too Busy to Diet

The Best Nutrition Guide for Busy People

Second Edition

Jacqueline King, MS, RDN, CDCES, FADA

Monica Joyce, MS, RDN, CDCES

Too Busy to Diet *The Best Nutrition Guide for Busy People*

ISBN 10: 978-1-7368323-0-1
Library of Congress Control Number: 2027075000

Manufactured in the United States of America

Book Cover and interior design by Amit Dey | amitdey2528@gmail.com

Additional copies of Too Busy to Diet can be purchased at Amazon.com in Kindle or paperback form at www.toobusytodietbook.com

Check out our website and blog: www.toobusytodietbook.com
Like us on Facebook: facebook.com/TooBusyToDiet
Follow us on Twitter: twitter.com /2busy2diet and Instagram.instagram.com/ 2busy2diet

* For bulk copies of this book for employers, member groups, health clubs, gyms, health related companies, health or fitness classes, businesses, educational classes or personal use, send an email to: dietking1@comcast.net

* For individualized nutrition plans, consultation, or lectures contact dietking1@comcast.net

TABLE OF CONTENTS

INTRODUCTION

"So much to do, so little time."

I f those words sound familiar, then this book is for you who packs a lot into a typical day. Never before has so much attention been focused on what we eat and how it impacts our health. The evidence is overwhelming that good nutrition and an exercise program can help you stay healthy and prevent disease. But how can we fit good nutrition and exercise into days packed with demands and responsibilities?

During our 80 years of combined nutrition experience we have counseled many individuals who struggle with incorporating healthy eating into their busy lives. Some may have had a recent medical diagnosis that requires diet and lifestyle changes. Others are concerned that their weight and lack of exercise may create health issues. Often, they are uncertain about how to begin making changes to improve their health.

From a personal perspective, Monica and I have collaborated on many projects over the years. Our book reflects many of the reoccurring nutrition concerns our clients face. During our own life experiences as working wives and moms (Monica- a single mom) we have experienced many of the same challenges. Now as grandparents we see many of our nutrition issues reflected in the lives of our busy adult children and their families. Juggling long work hours, children's demanding school and social/activity schedules can be a challenge for the most motivated parent and requires making healthy eating a priority.

In our book, we have addressed some of the barriers to healthy eating including processed and convenience foods, frequency of eating out, perceived lack of time to plan, shop and cook. Quick and efficient meal planning, shopping, and preparation remains a must.

We also retained our belief that healthy eating is enjoyable and when possible a family event. Our book also shares ways to handle special eating situations so one is confident dealing with a variety of eating situations.

Combining a busy lifestyle with healthy eating and exercise can be a challenge but is not impossible. Some of the same skills you use to achieve balance in your typical day can be used to balance your health and nutrition. Planning and organizing are the key ingredients, so the most overwhelming tasks become easy and routine.

Some of the questions you must ask yourself when beginning this book are:

- Am I ready to make changes to allow better eating habits for me and my family?
- Do I feel that making these changes will improve my health, allow me to feel better and give me more energy?
- Am I concerned that I will have difficulties overcoming challenges that healthy eating and exercising present?

After reading this book and making specific changes you should be used to the process. At this point:

- The practices presented have become a part of your daily life.
- You have incorporated the book's solutions to keep a routine.
- You have occasions when you lapse, but you able to get back on track easily.

You asked. We've listened. Over the years we've listened carefully to you – our patients, family and friends. We know living healthy is a top priority. We've tried not to nag or preach, knowing the time pressures and that your daily lives and health are intrinsically intertwined.

The patchwork of nutrition topics and easy food solutions reflect your concerns. Our topics will allow you to learn more about healthy eating, weight control, exercise, eating out, and meal planning and preparation. These also include easy meals and snacks, ways to shop more easily, and how to deal with high calorie beverages and popular foods.

Remember, healthy eating can be as easy as a quick trip to a local grocery store. Take some time out to plan a week of meals and snacks. Shopping shouldn't take more than 15 to 20 minutes, and cooking a meal no more than 30 minutes. Also included are easy meals and snacks, ways to shop more easily, and how to deal with high calorie beverages and popular foods.

No more "I'm too busy to diet. We hope you enjoy this book as much as we enjoyed writing it.

Bon Appétit!
Jackie and Monica

SECTION 1

CREATING A PLAN FOR HEALTHY EATING

HEALTHY EATING: EAT HEALTHY TO STAY HEALTHY

Let the food be the medicine and the medicine be the food"

— Hippocrates

The connection between the foods we eat and our health was recognized as far back as Hippocrates. Now there has never been a time when we have been so encouraged to take charge of our health by eating healthy and exercising more. Our diets should be made up of a variety of foods, emphasizing fruits, vegetables, and whole grains. There is no mystery to weight loss and management. The key strategy for losing weight has never changed: decrease calorie intake and increase physical activity. Drive-thru, convenience foods, and take-out foods are all around. Preparing fresh, less processed foods at home is done less and less. Fast and easy recipes are available, but it takes planning and shopping. If planned correctly, healthy eating can save you time, calories, and money.

When interviewed, individuals who spent much of their time "on the run" identified the availability of nutritious meals and snacks as a top priority. They acknowledged that traveling and eating out can interfere with eating healthy and maintaining a healthy body weight. Eating-on-the-go has led to an overweight epidemic we face today in America. We battle large portion sizes and calorie-dense foods that are easily accessible and often inexpensive; in most cases, we lose the battle and give in.

We are all moving less than ever. Many of us who have cars don't even think about walking to errands. Buses pick us up at the station and deposit us at our workplace, stealing the opportunity to walk. Some individuals complain of what's called "cubicilitis" or "computeritis", which in turn, limits our chances to move about during the workday. Down time is often spent at a computer or watching television. Too few of us meet the recommended 30 minutes or more of daily exercise. Because of this, every extra flight of stairs or 15 minutes of walking the family dog can really count.

CREATE A HEALTHY EATING PLAN

The path to healthy eating requires planning, shopping, and reading food labels to avoid eating whatever is in reach when in a rush. Choosing healthy foods requires a little effort. However, with practice, nutritious foods can quickly be incorporated into any lifestyle.

4 STEPS TO CREATING A HEALTHY MEAL PLAN

1. Plan: Spend a few minutes once a week to map out a week's worth of dinner menus. Menus can be repeated. As you become more proficient at meal planning, try planning a month of menus to avoid repetition. See Menu Planning Chapter.

2. Shop: Create a weekly shopping list. Busy professionals often complain they don't have nutritious foods in the house. Plan and use a list. A trip to the grocery store will take less than 30 minutes. When writing a grocery list, add some low-calorie convenience snacks and meals as "back-ups". This will save time, money, and calories when you are too tired to prepare a meal. See Shopping Chapter.

3. Read: Labels to avoid high-calorie foods. Some convenience foods have large amounts of sodium, fat, and calories that can be easily avoided by reading the label.

4. Cook: A simple yet nutritious meal can be prepared in less than thirty minutes. Cooking puts you in control of the quality or what you eat. Cooking can save calories and money, and often taste better than prepared foods. Purchase a cookbook with quick and easy menu ideas and recipes and get hooked on cooking. Check out our Easy Dinner Chapter.

Deciding to eat healthy and to exercise regularly is done by choice rather than chance. The first step in embarking on a healthy lifestyle or maintaining existing healthy lifestyle practices is recognizing its importance. Make a commitment to incorporate healthy choices and make good health a priority. The *January 2011 AND Journal* reports that diets high in vegetables, fruits, whole grains, poultry, fish, and low-fat dairy foods may affect the quality of life and mortality in the older adult populations. This study showed that the adults following this type of diet had more healthy years of life. Once the decision is made, it is important to stay the course. Weight loss or weight maintenance is not a week- long commitment, it is life-long. Consistency with a diet plan is crucial in order to obtain the desired results.

MY PLATE

The new icon, MyPlate, recently re-placed MyPyramid, used for over 20 years. MyPlate was introduced to help Americans make easier food choices to ensure that they are achieving a healthy diet.

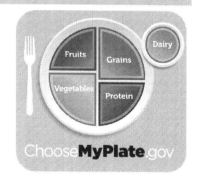

MyPlate can be found on the web-site: ChooseMyPlate.gov.

With the new website, the USDA emphasizes:

- Enjoying food but eating less
- Avoiding oversized portions
- Making half of your plate fruits and vegetables
- Drinking water instead of sugary drinks
- Switching to fat-free or low-fat milk
- Comparing the sodium content of foods
- Making half of your grains consumed whole grains
- Considering empty calories if you choose solid fats and added sugar

MyPlate is a new tool to assist in making daily food choices based on recommended servings of the five different food groups. Registered dietitians welcome this change since most dietitians have been using the plate-teaching tool for years. In both our practices, we are used to giving our patients paper plates to formulate their food plan easily. The MyPlate method continues to use the five-food group approach because most Americans continue to fail to get adequate amounts of fiber, the vitamins A, C, and E, and the minerals calcium, magnesium, and potassium in their daily diet. For this reason, MyPlate encourages a variety of foods, emphasizing a diet high in complex carbohydrates, low in sugar, and low in fats. Using MyPlate provides a diet adequate in vitamins and minerals. It also encourages a consumer to consider the portion of a serving when planning meals and snacks. MyPlate is divided into five food groups, with each group represented by a different color.

5 FOOD GROUPS

1. Grains (orange): Make half of your grains whole
2. Vegetables (green): Vary your veggies

3. Fruits (red): Focus on fruits

4. Dairy (blue): Get your calcium rich, low fat dairy choices

5. Meat and Beans (purple): Go lean with protein

In addition to a healthy diet, MyPlate also emphasizes the importance of physical activity. The incorporation of physical activity in every diet plan is extremely important in order to promote an overall healthy lifestyle.

My Plate's recommendations are based on the sex, age, and level of activity for each individual person. Go to choose my plate.gov to figure out how many calories you need and how many portions of each food group you should be receiving. This is also found on the first page of the Appendix. Under each food group, there is a reminder that if high fat items or sugar is added to the food choice, it is counted as empty calories from solid fats and added sugar. It has been recommended that empty calories should be limited to 10% of your calories each day. These new guidelines encourage individuals to maintain a desirable body weight. It highlights the importance of managing calories by focusing on portion control. MyPlate promotes weight loss by recommending that we lower our calories by eating less saturated fat and added sugars, as well as consuming less alcohol. Managing weight, getting adequate nutrition, and participating in a regular exercise program are all part of being heathy.

PLANT-BASED EATING

"Nothing will benefit human health and increase chances for survival of life on earth as much as the evolution to a vegetarian diet."

— *Albert Einstein*

Plant-Based Eating: Test your knowledge by answering True or False.

1. I am not a planted-based eater if I eat eggs or dairy.
2. As a plant-based eater, I will never be able to get adequate amounts of Vitamin B12 from my diet.
3. I do not have to worry about getting enough iron in my diet because I eat a lot of vegetables that are high in iron.
4. If I combine foods such as rice and beans or dairy and bread, I will be able to get complete protein in my diet.

Embracing plant-based eating whether it is flexitarian, vegetarian or vegan, has moved from the fringe and into the mainstream. People choose to follow a plant-based diet because:

- They don't like meat.
- They are concerned about animal welfare and the environment.

- They're concerned about their health
- They believe that a diet high in complex carbohydrates and fiber is healthier than one high in animal protein and saturated fat.
- It is part of their religion.

Whatever the reason, the health benefits of plant-based diets are undeniable. In 2016, the Academy of Nutrition and Dietetics stated that a vegetarian or vegan diet meets all the nutritional requirements for children, adults and pregnant or breast-feeding women. Plant-based eaters and vegans have a lower incidence of diabetes and fewer risk factors for cardiovascular disease, high blood pressure and cholesterol problems. Plant-based eaters also tend to eat more high-fiber foods. A recent study published in *Nutrients* compared satiety hormones in people following a plant-based diet versus a meat-based diet. The study found satiety hormones increased more in people on a plant-based diet and they reported greater satiety.

A vegetarian diet consists primarily of whole grains, fruits, vegetables, and legumes. Plant foods provides all the nutrients necessary for a balanced diet (with the exception of Vitamin B12) as well as variety and taste that can be adapted to fit any palate. Just be sure to include a variety of foods every day to ensure you are receiving the right vitamins, minerals, and essential amino acids.

PLANT-BASED TO VEGAN – WHAT'S RIGHT FOR YOU

Plant-based eating is a spectrum. Some people make some of their meals meatless. Others go all the way and become vegan, eating no animal products. Some choose to include eggs and dairy, while others include seafood or chicken.

Lacto-Ovo Vegetarian	• Includes cheese, eggs, milk, and grains.
Lacto-Plant-based Diets	• Includes cheese, milk, and yogurt. • Eliminates eggs and foods that contain eggs.
Vegan	• Eliminates eggs and dairy products, as well as foods that contain protein derivatives such as whey and casein. • Avoids honey since it comes from bees.
Semi-Plant-based (Flexitarian)	• Plant-based with the occasional fish, poultry, or meats.
Zen-Macrobiotic	• Limited to grains and very little fluid. • Not nutritionally adequate.
Macrobiotic	• Includes grains, legumes, nuts, and some vegetables. • Soy products are eaten frequently. • Fish may be included by some people. • Avoids dairy, eggs, and most fruit and vegetables from the nightshade family like tomatoes, potatoes, peppers, and eggplant.

BENEFITS AND CONCERNS

HEALTH AND WEIGHT MANAGEMENT BENEFITS:

1. Vegetarians are less likely to be extremely overweight.
2. Vegetarians are less likely to get cardiovascular disease, cancers, and gastrointestinal disorders.
3. Vegetarians tend to have lower blood pressure and LDL cholesterol and lower rates of hypertension and Type 2 Diabetes.

4. Vegetarian diets tend to be higher in fiber, magnesium, potassium, Vitamins C and E, folate, carotenoids, flavonoids and other phytochemicals.

5. Vegetarian diets tend to be lower in saturated fat and cholesterol.

Nutritional Concerns

Deficiencies can be avoided by choosing a wide variety of foods. The vitamins and minerals noted are in meats and can also be found in plant sources. Make sure your diet contains complete protein sources by combining whole grain breads, rice, and legumes.

Vitamin B12	
Purpose	Necessary for red blood cell maturation, nerve function, and DNA synthesis.
Symptoms	Anemia, dizziness, paleness, fatigue, neuropathy (nerve damage), and in more severe cases mental impairment, dementia and paranoia.
Sources	Lacto-ovo-vegetarians obtain B12 from dairy foods and eggs. Vegans need to eat food fortified with B12, such as cereal, seaweed, spirulina or take a B12 supplement.
	Breakfast cereals and Red Star Vegetarian Support Formula nutritional yeast provides. Good sources are milk, eggs, and cheese.
	Since these are animal products, vegans, and those following macrobiotic diets will need to get Vitamin B12 from enriched cereals and fortified soy products like vegetarian patties or taking a vitamin supplement.
	Multivitamins
Iron	
Purpose	Helps red blood cells carry oxygen throughout the body. It is also involved in the immune system and the synthesis of DNA.

Inhibits absorption	Calcium, fiber, phytates found in whole grains and dried beans, polyphenols found in tea, coffee, herbal teas and cocoa.
Enhances absorption	Vitamin C found in fruits and vegetables such as citrus, berries and bell peppers.
Symptoms	Some of the same symptoms as B12, deficiency, dizziness, paleness, fatigue, and shortness of breath are very common in women.
Recommended Intake	For plant eaters recommended intake is 1.8 times that of meat-eaters because the type of iron in plant foods is not easily absorbed.
Sources	Enriched whole-grain products like cereals and breads, dried peas and beans. Leafy green vegetables, dried fruits (raisins, apricots, prunes), and eggs.
Calcium	
Purpose	Key to building bone mass and density during puberty and maintaining bone health in adults. Calcium is also required for nerve transmission and muscle regulation, especially in the heart.
Symptoms	Low dietary intake may contribute to decreased bone mass. If diet is low in both vitamin D and calcium, it can contribute to osteomalacia or softening of the bones. Plant-eaters tend to have high intakes of calcium often higher than those of meat eaters. Vegans tend to have lower calcium intakes with a 30% higher risk for bone fraction.
Sources	Soy milk, rice milk and breakfast cereal. Dairy products are the best source of calcium. Dark green leafy vegetables, such as spinach, collard greens, turnips, kale, bok choy, Chinese cabbage, and broccoli. Tofu enriched with calcium.

Vitamin D	
Purpose	Helps maintain calcium levels, contributing to healthy bones and teeth. Also, more than 50 genes are known to be regulated by vitamin D.
Symptoms	Rickets in children and osteomalacia in adults. Calcitriol is the active form of vitamin D in the body. Our bodies convert cholesterol in the skin into vitamin D using the sun's ultra-violet light. People living in northern climates, those with dark skin, and those who use large amounts of sunscreen could be deficient in Vitamin D. Also vegan and macrobiotic diets that do not include fortified food or supplements may not supply enough Vitamin D.
Sources	The sun, food, and drinks fortified with Vitamin D such milk, orange juice, rice drinks, cereal, margarines, many soy products and some yogurts and cheese.

Herring, sardines, salmon, shrimp, and some mushrooms.

If sunlight is limited use a Vitamin D supplement. |
| **Zinc** | |
| Purpose | Important in growth and development, immune response, neurological function and reproduction. |
| Symptoms | Vegans may need zinc supplementation because plant staples are most of their diet.

Phytic acid, found in plants and other whole grain products, reduce zinc absorption. If yeast is used to leaven whole grain bread, zinc becomes available for absorption by the body.

Mild deficiency can impair physical and neurological development and inability to fight infection especially in children. |
| Sources | Leavened whole grain bread products, shellfish, nuts, and legumes, eggs, dairy, cheese, soy products, beans (white, kidney, chickpeas), pumpkin seeds and yogurt. |

Omega-3 Fatty Acids

Purpose	Fatty acids eicosapentaenoic acid (EPA) and docosahexaenoic acid (DHA) are omega-3 (n-3) fatty acids known for their important role in cardiovascular health and eye and brain development. Vegans tend to have lower levels of EPA and DHA.
	Vegetarian diets are usually high in omega-6 fatty acids but may be low in n-3 fatty acids.
Sources	DHA-fortified soy milk and breakfast bars, fatty fish, such as bluefish tuna, canned and wild salmon, mackerel, sardines, fish oil supplements, walnuts.

Iodine

Purpose	Essential trace minerals concentrated in the thyroid gland are key to synthesis of thyroid hormones.
Symptoms	Goiter, which is a large visible lump on the neck, caused by the increase in Thyroid-Stimulating Hormone (TSH) This is also a symptom of iodine excess.
	Plant-based diets can be low in iodine. Those who don't use iodized salt or sea vegetables may be at risk for iodine deficiency.
Sources	Depends upon the soil where food is grown. Mountainous areas and river deltas are usually deficient in iodine.
	Seafood and seaweed, milk, iodized salt, (not present in sea salt).

Protein

Purpose	Protein helps make up the structure and function of our body; DNA, cells, nerves, skin, muscles, hair etc.
Symptoms	Change in hair color, hair loss, fatigue, and fluid retention. Since B vitamins are part of most protein products, anemia may also result.

Recommended Intake	A plant-based diet that includes eggs and dairy products will usually provide enough protein in the diet. When avoiding meat, it is important to consume foods containing complete protein.
Sources	Milk, eggs, nuts, and beans are sources of protein. By eating a variety of plant proteins over the course of a day all the essential amino acids can be provided.
	Soy is the best known of the plant proteins. It contains all the essential amino acids, making it a complete protein. In fact, soy is the only food with plant protein that is equal in quality to the protein found in meat and eggs.
	Tempeh is a soy protein that also provides fiber, B vitamins, and iron.
	Its mild flavor makes it compatible with many dishes such as casseroles, stir frys, and chili.
	Soy yogurt is a portable soy product that can make a great snack and is high in nutrition.
	Tofu or bean curd is a good source of protein and calcium. It most often is an ingredient in "meat analogs" also known as meat substitutes and veggie burgers.
	Be sure to read labels to find out.

Plant-Based Eaters ON THE MOVE!

Following a plant-based diet is easier than ever. Product availability has grown with the increased focus on plant-based eating, the environment, and sustainability. More and more fortified foods, including breakfast cereals, juices, and soy milk, are appearing on grocery store shelves.

More plant-based and vegan fresh and frozen meals are available in grocery stores, restaurants, and fast-food establishments that have made plant-based eating an easier option.

PLANT-BASED EATING ON THE GO

1. **Grocery Shopping**: The variety of foods offered at grocery stores is greater than ever. Frozen food sections now offer vegan meals. Look for whole grains and meals lower in sodium. Two reliable brands are Amy's and Dr. Praeger's. Trader Joe's also offers vegan options.

2. **Quick Meals**: Boxed mixes such as rice pilaf, risotto, quinoa, rice dishes, couscous, and vegetable chili, can turn into a healthy vegan meal in no time. Add a vegetable or salad and fruit to make it complete. Many brands also offer meatless options that include fish or dairy.

3. **Fast Foods**: Many fast food restaurants have meatless alternatives that can fit easily into a vegetarian diet. For instance, Wendy's serves baked potatoes with cheese and broccoli. Other meatless meals on the run can include cheese pizza with a salad, veggie pizza, grilled veggie sandwiches, veggie burgers, or a bean burrito. Be aware of sodium and fat when choosing from fast food restaurants. Try to balance the day with low-fat, low-sodium foods at other meals.

4. **Restaurants**: If a restaurant does not offer plant-based items, you can often create a meal by asking if the chef could eliminate meat fillings or toppings. Or, try choosing a variety of meatless appetizers or side dishes. But if you're eating a vegan diet, check to make sure that soups and sauces are made with vegetable broth and not chicken broth.

5. **Ethnic foods**: Some ethnic dishes (especially Italian, Mexican, Indian, and Chinese) can be easily incorporated into a plant-based eating style. Vegetable lasagna, cheese ravioli, and manicotti stuffed with spinach and cheese are plant-based Italian meals. Bean tacos or burritos, cheese quesadillas, and vegetable fajitas are popular meatless Mexican foods.

Mediterranean foods including falafel, hummus, tahini, and chickpeas can make easy meals. Try Moroccan dishes, e.g. (fava beans with red lentils). Egyptian koshari (rice, lentils and macaroni) can also make great meals.

6. **Travel and banquets**: Plant-based meals usually can be reserved. Most banquets set aside vegetarian dishes "just in case." International flights and domestic flights offering meals also offer plant-based meals. That can be requested when reserving your ticket.

PLAN TO SUCCEED

1. **Warm up with a few meatless meals.** Switch to complex carbohydrates like whole-wheat bread and pasta and brown rice. Replace one meal per day with a meatless meal. Choose beans or eggs instead of meat. For example, try cheese ravioli with marinara sauce, a salad, and whole-grain bread or a hearty bean soup with a whole-grain roll and salad.

2. **Variety and balance.** Mix and match from your four vegetarian food groups: grains, legumes, vegetables, and fruit. Choose a variety of fruits, vegetables, and low-fat dairy to get a mix of vitamins and minerals. Replace white all-purpose flour with 100% whole-wheat flour. Make burgers out of tofu, beans, and brown rice.

3. **Plant-based recipes:** Many websites that provide plant-based recipes. Practice fixing different foods and have a friend over to try them out. Experiment and see if simple substitutions can turn your favorite dishes into vegetarian go-to meals.

4. **Quick plant-based** Cooking can be quick and easy if you plan. If you haven't much time, prepare some pasta, which cooks up in minutes. Add a pesto sauce or sauté fresh tomatoes with onion and garlic for a quick sauce. Add Parmesan cheese

and a salad. Try tofu in a stir-fry. Add soybeans or tofu to chili or casseroles. You can also try black bean or chickpea veggie burgers, or beet or mushroom-based burger patties.

5. **Back up foods.** Stock your freezer with cheese ravioli, tortellini, and gnocchi. Add a salad, bread, and vegetables for a complete meal.

6. **Soups.** Keep a variety of meatless canned soups on hand. Many soups contain both legumes and vegetables. But watch the sodium content. Or make your own soup using low-sodium or no-salt added canned beans, broth and frozen vegetables. Freeze leftovers for later.

7. **Snacks.** Some nutritious options include nuts (especially almonds, walnuts, and soy nuts), fruit, yogurt, granola bars, pretzels, carrot sticks, apple and nut butters, grapes and berries, popcorn, and granola. Make your own trail mix from soy nuts, raisins, dried cranberries, almonds, and apricots. *

* Soy snack ideas from *The Soy Connection*, Spring 2011

Vegan
MY ∧PLATE

Nutrition Tips:

*Choose mostly whole grains.
*Eat a variety of foods from each of the food groups.
*Adults age 70 and younger need 600 IU of vitamin D daily.
 Sources include fortified foods (such as some soymilks) or a vitamin D supplement.
*Sources of iodine include iodized salt (3/8 teaspoon daily) or
 an iodine supplement (150 micrograms).
* See www.vrg.org for recipes and more details.

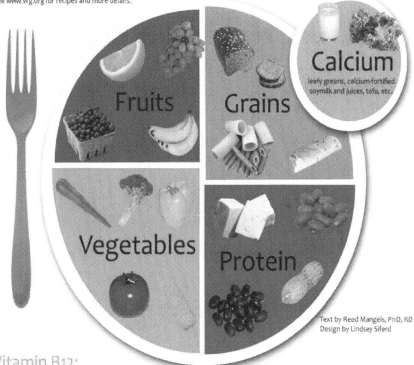

Calcium
leafy greens, calcium-fortified soymilk and juices, tofu, etc.

Fruits

Grains

Vegetables

Protein

Text by Reed Mangels, PhD, RD
Design by Lindsey Siferd

Vitamin B12:

Vegans need a reliable source of vitamin B12. Eat daily a couple of servings of fortified foods
such as B12-fortified soymilk, breakfast cereal, meat analog, or Vegetarian Support Formula nutritional yeast.
Check the label for fortification. If fortified foods are not eaten daily,
you should take a vitamin B12 supplement (25 micrograms daily).

Note:

Like any food plan, this should only serve as a general guide for adults.
The plan can be modified according to your own personal needs. This is not personal
medical advice. Individuals with special health needs should consult a registered
dietitian or a medical doctor knowledgeable about vegan nutrition.

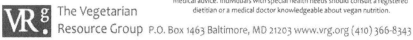

VRg. The Vegetarian
Resource Group P.O. Box 1463 Baltimore, MD 21203 www.vrg.org (410) 366-8343

PROTEIN CONTENT OF SELECT PLANT FOODS

Food	Amount	Protein	Protein (grams) (g)/100 calories
(Tempeh	1 cup	41	9.3
Seitan	3 oz	31	22.1
Soybeans (edamame), cooked	1 cup	29	9.6
Lentils, cooked	1 cup	18	7.8
Black beans, cooked	1 cup	15	6.7
Kidney beans, cooked	1 cup	13	6.4
Veggie Burger	1 patty	13	13.0
Chickpeas, cooked	1 cup	12	4.2
Veggie baked beans	1 cup	12	5.0
Pinto Beans, cooked	1 cup	12	5.7
Black-eyed peas, cooked	1 cup	11	6.2
Tofu, firm	4 oz	11	11.7
Lima beans, cooked	1 cup	10	5.7
Quinoa, cooked	1 cup	9	3.5
Tofu, regular	4 oz	9	10.6
Bagel	1 med/3 oz	9	3.9
Peas, cooked	1 cup	9	6.4
Textured Vegetable Protein (TVP), cooked	1/2 cup	8	6.4
Peanut butter	2 tbsp.	8	4.3
Veggie Dog	1 link	8	13.3
Spaghetti, cooked	1 cup	8	3.7
Almonds	1/4 cup	8	3.7
Soy yogurt, plain	6 oz	6	4.0

Bulgur, cooked	1 cup	6	3.7
Sunflower seeds	1/4 cup	6	3.3
Whole-wheat Bread	2 slices	5	3.9
Cashews	1/4 cup	5	2.7
Almond butter	2 tbsp.	5	2.4
Brown rice, cooked	1 cup	5	2.1
Spinach, cooked	1 cup	5	13.0
Broccoli, cooked	1 cup	4	6.8
Potato	1 med/6 oz	4	2.7

Sources: USDA Nutrient Database for Standard Reference, Release 18, 2005 and manufacturers' information

The recommendation for protein for adult male vegans is around 56-70 grams per day; for adult female vegans it is around 46-58 grams per day.

DAIRY AND NON-DAIRY MILK ALTERNATIVES

Type of milk	Serving size	Calories	Carbs (g)	Protein (g)	Fat (g)
Almond	1 cup	40	2	1	3
Coconut	1 cup	552	13	5.5	57
Hemp	1 cup	72	3	3.8	5
Rice	1 cup	120	33	3.8	5.5
Soy	1 cup	100	8	7	4
Cow, 2%	1 cup	120	12	8	5

Choose those fortified with calcium and vitamin D to achieve your daily requirement. See the Calcium Chapter.

Answers to Plant-Based Diet Questions:

1. False. A Lacto-ovo plant-based diets include eggs and dairy.
2. False. Although more difficult, it is possible to obtain adequate amounts of B12 if you eat plant-based sources of B12 or take a supplement.
3. False. It is difficult to get enough iron through vegetables. They are not a good source of iron, and the iron they do contain is not well absorbed. Iron fortified cereals, other iron-fortified foods, or supplements should be consumed.
4. True

MEDITERRANEAN WAY

"You don't have to cook fancy or complicated masterpieces - just good food from fresh ingredients."

— Julia Child

The Mediterranean Diet has evolved over thousands of years, shaped by a rich and multifaceted ethnic population with diverse cultural and religious practices. The people have embraced a similar eating pattern that uses seasonal, local foods to create dishes that are not only healthy but taste great. This diet includes an abundance of plant foods including vegetables, fruits, legumes, whole grains, and nuts. The diet is rich in vitamins, minerals, antioxidants, polyphenols, and fiber. It also contains several sources of omega-3 fatty acids such as fatty fish, greens such as kale and spinach, and walnuts, which help protect against heart disease. In fact, there is a balance of both omega-6 to omega-3 polyunsaturated fatty acids.

Scientists believe omega-6 fats tend to be proinflammatory while omega-3 fats have more anti-inflammatory action. The American diet leans heavily toward omega-6 fats, leading to more negative health consequences such as obesity, cardiovascular disease, fatty liver disease, and other diseases linked to inflammation.

Studies from the last few decades have shown that despite a moderate to high intake of salt, fat, and alcohol (red wine), residents of the region have a much lower rate of cardiovascular disease than people in the United States. The Lyon Heart Study in

1998 found a 70% lower incidence of nonfatal repeat heart attacks in people who followed a Mediterranean diet versus those on a low-fat diet that was high in polyunsaturated fat. A study in the *New England Journal of Medicine* in 2008 found that people who followed a Mediterranean diet lost more weight. A study in The *British Medical Journal* in the same year showed a reduced risk of dying from cancer and cardiovascular disease, as well as less risk for Parkinson's and Alzheimer's diseases. A study reported in the *American Journal of Clinical Nutrition* in 2013 found that menopausal women who ate a Mediterranean style diet reported that they were 20 percent less likely to have hot flashes and night sweats than women who ate diets higher in fat and sugar. A healthy gut microbiome has also been associated with the diet.

BREAKING DOWN THE MEDITERRANEAN DIET

Fruits, Vegetables, and Whole Grains: Plant foods rule the plate. Some meals are completely meatless. Sauces are often made with yogurt, fresh vegetables, and herbs. Fruit is more likely the end to a meal instead of dessert and can be used as a between meal snack.

Oils, Fats, and Meats: Total fat in the diet is 25% to 35% of calories. Saturated fat is about 8% or less of total calories. Over half the fat in the diet is from healthy monounsaturated fat. These fats include olive oil and nuts.

- Extra-virgin and virgin olive oils: The least processed oils containing the highest amounts of polyphenols and antioxidants.
- Red meats: Eaten less often than fish and poultry, lowering intake of saturated fat and cholesterol.
- Fish: Eaten two to three times per week. Good choices include tuna, salmon, mackerel, herring, albacore tuna, and trout because of their higher content of omega-3 fatty acids.

Portions: It's not just choosing healthy foods, but also managing portions. A portion of protein is generally about 4 ounces cooked. When visiting any Mediterrean country, one is often surprised at the smaller portion sizes. Snacking is rare, and coffee or espresso breaks usually are not accompanied by a dessert or snack.

Seasonings: Fresh herbs and spices are used more often than salt.

Natural Foods: Processed foods and fast food are not a part of everyday life.

Wine: Moderate amounts of wine, particularly red wine, is enjoyed with meals.

WHAT MAKES THIS A GOOD DIET?

The Mediterrean diet is great because it is not a diet at all. It is a pattern of eating that is plant-based, local and seasonal. It includes a variety of quality foods that provide the right nutrients in the right amounts. The diet is high in complex carbohydrates, making it naturally high in fiber, includes a greater proportion of healthy unsaturated fats, and is rich in a variety of nutrients. The Mediterrean diet includes:

- Fruits and vegetables.
- Whole-grain breads, pastas, rice, and cereals.
- Beans, nuts, and seeds.
- Foods low in saturated and trans fats, foods which have been shown to increase cholesterol levels and contribute to heart disease.
- Fish, poultry, and dairy are the main sources of animal protein and are used sparingly.
- Red meat is eaten only occasionally.

High amounts of monosaturated fat from olive oil, olives, and canola oil:

* Olive oil has beneficial anti-inflammatory properties.

● Monounsaturated fat has been shown to reduce LDL (bad) cholesterol levels.

High amounts of omega-3 fatty acids:

● Sources include fish, olive oil, and nuts (especially walnuts).

● Omega-3 fatty acids have been shown to lower triglycerides, improving blood vessel health.

Moderate intake of wine:

● Red wine has been shown to increase HDL (good) cholesterol.

● It is a good source of the phytochemical resveratrol, which has been shown to prevent clotting and plaque formation in arteries.

● Limit to 5 ounces (1 serving) per day for women and 10 ounces (2 servings) per day for men.

Fad diets come and go because they have no roots or science to back them. Yet the Mediterranean diet and the lifestyle that accompanies it has been linked to good health for ages. Unlike others, the Mediterranean diet includes a variety of healthy foods that are enjoyable and sustain person and planet.

HOW CAN I ADOPT THIS DIET?

1. Try fish and poultry recipes. Baking, broiling, and grilling are fast and require little preparation. Cooking at home can take less time than eating a meal out.

2. Find a handful of easy-to-prepare recipes. Try Alexander Lindberg, MD, Eating the Greek Way or Amy Riolo, The Mediterranean Diabetes Cookbook: A Flavorful, Low -Fat, Heart-Healthy Approach to Cooking.

3. Limit red meat to 3 servings per week.

4. Use herbs and spices to enhance flavor and less salt.

5. Make pasta dishes for a fast and easy meal. A meatless sauce can be prepared in minutes by sautéing fresh tomatoes, onions, and other vegetables in olive oil. Use seasonal vegetables to vary your recipe and keep meals interesting.

6. Use olive oil when cooking and on salads and vegetables.

7. Cook fresh or frozen vegetables for a side dish.

8. Finish off your meal with fresh fruit and low-fat cheese. This will help you cut back on added sugar from desserts.

9. Try a handful of walnuts or almonds as a snack or sprinkle on a dish.

10. Check with your doctor about adding a glass of red wine with a meal.

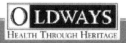

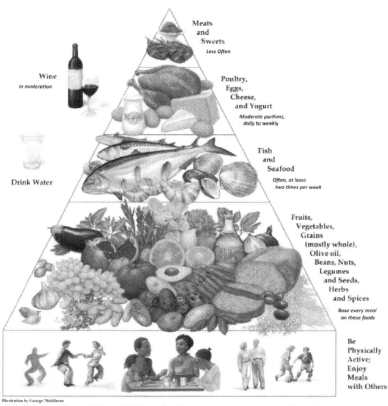

Illustration by George Middleton

© 2009 Oldways Preservation and Exchange Trust   www.oldwayspt.org

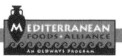

VITAMINS: NUTRIENTS FOR OPTIMAL HEALTH

"Adam and Eve ate the first vitamins, including the package."

— E.R. Squibb

Vitamin and Mineral Supplement Questions: Test your knowledge by answering True or False to the questions below.

1. A vitamin supplement is probably not necessary if you are eating a variety of foods
2. Taking vitamins can substitute for eating a healthy diet
3. Vitamins can be important for those with some diseases, poor appetite, pregnancy, or plant-based eating
4. Doubling your daily vitamin intake will make you healthier
5. Taking single vitamin and mineral supplements is better than taking a multivitamin with added minerals
6. Natural vitamins are superior to synthetic vitamins

VITAMIN AND MINERAL SUPPLEMENTS

Vitamins and minerals are building blocks of life and health. And getting them from natural, whole foods in most cases is best.

A study published in the Journal of the American College of Cardiology showed that the most commonly used supplements—vitamin D and C, multivitamins, and calcium did not help prevent heart disease, heart attack, stroke, or premature death. In this study, the supplements didn't hurt, but the takers gained nothing. The study's lead author stated that there is no harm in using supplements, but there is no apparent advantage either. The study did show that folic acid alone or with other B vitamins may reduce heart disease or stroke. The best that researchers and dietitians have to offer concerning supplements is to eat a well-balanced diet to obtain the optimal levels of vitamins and minerals. That's not to say vitamins and mineral supplements don't have a place next to your healthy plate in certain situations. Some health professionals may recommend vitamins or minerals for individuals at increased risk of developing nutrient deficiencies including those who are:

- Pregnant
- Lactating
- Dieting
- Perimenopausal
- Elderly
- Have chronic diseases
- A history of alcohol, drug, or tobacco use
- Taking certain medications
- Experiencing stress
- Skipping meals
- Making less than optimal food choices

Vitamin and mineral supplements use first became popular in the early 1900s, a time when it was difficult to obtain a wide assortment of fruits and vegetables year-round. Since then, many of the most common nutrient deficiencies have been addressed through enriching and fortifying foods. It is highly unlikely for anyone to be seriously deficient today unless there is an underlying medical condition.

Advertising may say otherwise. But remember, the primary purpose of advertising is to generate revenue for the company, not necessarily to improve your health. Beware of anyone selling supplements. Their motivation is their own financial gain, not your health. Registered dietitians are the best source of information; they can evaluate your diet and let you know if there are any deficiencies that need to be corrected by either diet or supplements. They can also help you boost your vitamin and mineral intake through food first, which will ultimately be better for your body and your credit card statement.

VITAMINS

Vitamins fall into two categories, water-soluble and fat-soluble. Water-soluble vitamins usually help regulate metabolism and the production and release of energy, aid the production of red blood cells, and strengthen the immune system.

They also serve as antioxidants. The water-soluble vitamins (except Vitamin C) also help enzymes function in the body and protect cells from damage done by free radicals within the body.

The nine water-soluble vitamins are lost easily when food is overcooked. They mix easily in the blood, and the excess is excreted in the urine. Only small amounts are stored in the body, so it's important to get them in your daily diet to avoid deficiencies.

Fat-soluble vitamins ensure proper cell growth, healthy vision, strong bone development, and antioxidant protection. The fat-soluble vitamins -- A, D, E, and K -- are absorbed with fat from food. They can accumulate in toxic amounts in the body because they are not excreted in urine like water-soluble vitamins. Too much vitamin K can be toxic to individuals on anticoagulant medications when taken in large amounts long-term. Vitamins A and D have also been shown to be toxic with doses at 15 and 5 times the RDA, respectively.

Recent research is showing that one vitamin that should not be missed is Vitamin D. The adequate amounts of the sunshine vitamin has been linked to a reduction in heart attacks, a reduction in at least a dozen types of cancer, and improved absorption of calcium. Find more on vitamin D in the Calcium Chapter.

Large doses of Vitamin E have not been found to be toxic. However, taking amounts greater than 800 IU per day have not been found to be beneficial. And large doses of Vitamin E can cause complications for those taking blood thinners, antiplatelet drugs, anti-inflammatory drugs (NSAIDs), or those who have bleeding disorders.

When it comes to vitamins -- and minerals as well – more is not better, and in fact can be harmful. Megavitamin therapy, the use of supplements in amounts that exceed the recommended daily allowance (RDA) by 10 times or more, is unnecessary and can be expensive and harmful.

MINERALS

The role of minerals in the body are similar to vitamins, including serving as cofactors, releasing and making energy, acting as antioxidants, and regulating metabolism. And they do even more work such as maintaining acid-base balance and aiding muscle contraction and nerve conduction. The amount of minerals absorbed depends on the other nutrients eaten in the meal, the form of the mineral, and whether it is chemically bound to other nutrients.

Just like some vitamins, large doses of certain minerals, even as little as a few times the RDA, can be dangerous if they accumulate in your tissues. They can actually cause a secondary deficiency of other minerals. For example, iron taken in large amounts can cause constipation, stomach and gastrointestinal upset, and can accumulate in the liver, pancreas, and other organs, causing a condition called hemosiderosis. Large amounts of selenium can cause nervous system disorders, liver problems, or kidney disorders. Large doses of zinc can cause a copper deficiency because the two minerals compete for absorption in the small intestine.

Just as megavitamin therapy can cause problems, mega amounts of minerals -- anywhere from 10 to 1,000 times the RDA -- for long periods of time can be detrimental. With the exception of iron, minerals are generally absorbed better with meals. Iron, however; is absorbed much better on an empty stomach but can cause nausea.

Water-Soluble Vitamins

- Vitamin C
- The B Vitamins:
  - Thiamin (B1)
  - Riboflavin (B2)
  - Niacin (B3)
  - Pantothenic acid (B5)
  - Pyridoxine (B6)
  - Biotin (B7)
  - Folic acid (B9)
  - Cyanocobalamin (B12)

MEGA-DOSE DANGERS

- Excessive vitamin A or niacin intake can cause liver damage.
- Excessive vitamin C or zinc intake can reduce the immune response and increase the risk of kidney stones.
- Excessive vitamin B6 intake can cause irreversible nerve damage
- Excessive vitamin B5 or pantothenic acid can cause diarrhea.

Supplement manufacturers don't have to prove their products are safe, actually have any benefits or even contain the labeled ingredients and only those ingredients before they sell them online or in stores. Mislabeled, inadequately labeled and contaminated products are a hazard and not as rare as they should be. Regulators only step in after a product has been for sale and consumers have filed complaints or been harmed. Another reason to go food first for nutrients.

Added calories are another hazard. Vitaminwater by the Coca Cola Company touts improved physical and mental well-being. But it has over 33 grams of added sugar and 132 calories in a 20-ounce bottle

HELPFUL VITAMIN-MINERAL TERMS:

- **Buffered vitamins** - Some vitamins (in particular, vitamin C) are acidic and can irritate the digestive tract if taken in mega-doses. Buffered vitamins have a compound added to neutralize the acid and make them less irritating.

- **Chelated minerals**-These minerals are attached to another substance to enhance absorption. However, the acid in the stomach breaks this attachment. These minerals are attached to another substance to enhance absorption. However, the acid in the stomach breaks this attachment. Chelated forms of iron fumerate and zinc gluconate have been found to be less irritating to the stomach and intestine, reducing stomach upsets and constipation when taken in large amounts. The chelated form of chromium (chromium picolinate) is also very well absorbed.

- **Chewable vitamins** - Chewable vitamins are an easy way to encourage children (who may not yet be able to swallow pills) to take a multivitamin. However, since children's multivitamins taste like candy, their vitamin consumption should be carefully monitored and bottles kept out of their reach. A child's smaller size can increase susceptibility to vitamin toxicity. Plus exposing tooth enamel to vitamin C in chewable vitamins can increase the risk of cavities.

- **Natural, Organic, or Synthetic Vitamins** - "Natural" or "organic" vitamins have been promoted as providing increased absorption and health benefits. These products make false or exaggerated claims and are usually more expensive. There is no scientific evidence showing that the body uses natural or organic vitamins and minerals better than synthetic forms. The body does not recognize a natural or organic vitamin or mineral supplement any differently than it would a synthetic form.

- **Time-Released Supplements** - It was originally thought this would benefit the body by having vitamins and minerals available to the body for longer periods of time. But the nutrients in time-released supplements are often more poorly absorbed. Some nutrients have also been found to be more toxic to certain organs when in time-released forms. Time-released supplements should be monitored or avoided if possible.

Answers to Vitamin and Mineral Questions:

1. True.
2. False. A vitamin supplement may be taken in addition to a healthy diet. No vitamin supplement can replace the nutrients and fiber in healthy foods.
3. True. In cases of stress, increased energy needs, or lack of consumption of all food groups, a vitamin supplement is important to avoid deficiencies.
4. False. As long as you meet the RDA for vitamins and minerals, there is no need to double your daily intake.
5. False. Neither form is better than the other; however, if you are deficient in a specific nutrient, a single supplement may be more beneficial. On the other hand, if you want to ensure

adequate vitamin and mineral intake throughout the day, a multivitamin would be more beneficial to you.

6. False. There is no evidence supporting this claim. All vitamins are recognized the same in the body no matter the source.

USDA DAILY AMOUNTS

Fat Soluble Vitamins	RDA Females (31-50)	RDA Males (31-50)
Vitamin A**	900 mcg RAE	700 mcg RAE
Beta-carotene**	None	None
Vitamin D**	5 mcg	5 mcg
Vitamin E	15 mg a-TE	15 mg a-TE
Vitamin K	120 mcg	90 mcg
Water Soluble Vitamins	**RDA Males (31-50)**	**RDA Females (31-50)**
Vitamin B1	1.2 mg	1.1 mg
Vitamin B2	1.3 mg	1.1 mg
Niacin	16 mg NE	14 mg NE
Vitamin B6	1.3 mg	1.3 mg
Vitamin B12	2.4 mcg	2.4 mcg
Folic Acid	400 mcg DFE	400 mcg DFE
Biotin	30 mce	30 mcg
Pantothenic Acid	5 mg	5 mg
Vitamin C	90 mg	75 mg

Minerals RDA	Males (31-50)	RDA Females (31-50)
Calcium**	1000 mg	1000 mg
Chromium	35 mcg	25 mcg
Copper**	900 mcg	900 mcg
Iron**	8 mg	18 mg
Magnesium	420 mg	320 mg
Manganese	2.3 mg	1.8 mg
Molybdenum	45 mcg	45 mcg
Selenium	55 mcg	55 mcg
Zinc**	11 mg	8 mg

**These vitamins and minerals can be dangerous in excess amounts.

Review the following charts to see where you can obtain vitamins from your food:

Vitamin A

- Tomatoes
- Carrots
- Sweet Potatoes
- Pumpkin

Vitamin C

- Oranges
- Red/Green Peppers
- Brussel Sprouts
- Papaya

Vitamin E

- Almonds
- Sunflower Oil
- Asparagus
- Peanuts

Vitamin D

- Herring
- Salmon
- Fortified Milk
- Sardines

Vitamin K

- Spinach
- Iceberg Lettuce
- Broccoli
- Cabbage

Thiamine

- Fortified Cereal
- Pork Chops
- Ham
- Sunflower Seeds

Riboflavin

- Beef Liver
- Fortified Cereal
- Milk
- Yogurt

Vitamin B6

- Potato
- Banana
- White Rice
- Chicken

Folate

- Black-eyed Peas
- Lentils
- Spinach
- Fortified Milk

Vitamin B12

- Beef Liver
- Clams, Tuna, Trout, Oysters, Crab
- Fortified yeast, cereal, and milk and dairy products then add Eggs

Iron Rich foods

- Red meat
- Dark turkey meat
- Beans and legumes
- Pumpkin seeds
- Broccoli
- Quinoa
- Spirulina
- Dark Chocolate
- Spinach
- Tofu

*Consuming vitamin C rich foods helps with iron absorption

BRAIN-GUT DIET CONNECTION

New research shows that food and brain health is affected more than we thought. The Anxiety and Depression Association of America reports that anxiety is the most common mental illness in America, and it affects 18% of the population. Depression affects 6.7% of the population each year, and 15% of adults will experience depression during their lifetime. Nutrition is not a cure but may play a part in managing symptoms

In September 2018, the *World Journal of Psychiatry* published "Antidepressant foods: An Evidence Based Nutrient Profiling System for Depression." One of its authors, Dr. Drew Ramsey highlighted 12 antidepressant nutrients: folate, iron, long-chain omega-3 fatty acids, magnesium, potassium, selenium, thiamin, vitamin A, vitamin B6, vitamin B12, vitamin C, and zinc. Check the Vitamin Chapter, for foods high in these vitamins and iron, and the Cholesterol Chapter for foods high in omega-3 fatty acids. Research has found that these nutrients may help in the prevention and treatment of depressive disorders.

The highest scoring foods were oysters, mussels, seafoods, organ meats, leafy greens, lettuces, peppers, and cruciferous vegetables.

A Mediterranean style eating pattern, with its high amount of omega-3 fatty acids was found to be important in helping maintain brain health.

Research has found that certain vegetables stimulate serotonin release in the body, which reduces our vulnerability to stress. Unfortunately, Americans are not consuming the recommended five vegetable and fruit servings daily. A Mediterranean diet usually has about nine vegetable and fruit servings recommended.

Heart-healthy fats, especially omega-3 fatty acids can improve mood. Salmon, tuna, and bass contain omega-3 fatty acids, which are also present in some plant foods such as flax seed and chia seeds. Monounsaturated fats found in avocado, olive oil, and nuts are also helpful in elevating mood. It is also important to have adequate complex carbohydrates like whole grains to go along with healthy fats and vegetables. Individuals often complain of headaches and related symptoms from stress. But those symptoms could be from the brain not getting enough of the carbohydrates it needs to function properly.

To get enough carbohydrates for proper brain function and mood balance, it is important not to skip meals. Healthy fats are also important in allowing the hunger hormone ghrelin to create that feeling of fullness. There are many psychiatrists that feel that the gut-brain connection is the key to managing anxiety and depression. Dr. Uma Naidoo, a psychiatry professor at Harvard Medical School, culinary instructor at Cambridge School of Culinary Arts, and director of nutritional psychiatry at Massachusetts General Hospital feels strongly that this connection plays a part in proper brain function. She states that an imbalance in our gut-brain connection causes inflammation and disrupts the balance of the hormones and neurotransmitters in the brain. She has added nutrition to her therapy because she sees a connection between the medications she prescribes and the foods that patients eat. This is important because many of the medications used for anxiety and depression cause weight gain. Managing weight is crucial to improving mental and physical health.

Dr. Naidoo also includes therapy to improve sleep, exercise, and mindfulness. Along with Dr. Ramsey, assistant clinical professor of psychiatry at Columbia University, Dr. Naidoo has collaborated with chef David Bouley, the chef behind the New York restaurant Bouley at Home and Bouley Test Kitchen. Together they have worked with doctors to educate medical professionals and cooks to promote the connection between food and physical wellness. They feel strongly that eating fermented foods brings "good bacteria" or probiotics to the digestive system, which helps ease anxiety in the brain. Fermented foods include:

- Kefir
- Cultured milk and yogurt.
- Wine
- Beer
- Cider
- Tempeh
- Miso
- Kimchi
- Sauerkraut

The intersection of the sciences of nutrition and brain health is just beginning to evolve. These doctors and chefs are paving the way. More dietitians, nurses, and other health professionals are incorporating nutrition into their therapy. Mental health and nutritional specialists are recommending that "Nutritional Psychiatry" become part of mental health clinical practice and part of medical school curriculum.

SECTION 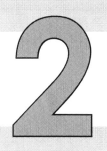2

LOSING AND
MAINTAINING WEIGHT

WEIGHING YOUR BEST

"To eat is a necessity, but to eat intelligently is an art."

— La Rouchefoucauld

Forget about those commercials promising fast and easy weight loss. Losing weight is difficult and takes time. Maintaining weight loss is an even bigger challenge. Changing our environment as well as what, when and how much we eat can be a struggle. Fortunately, we now have a better understanding of the link between obesity and genetics and how they affect health. We know there are hundreds of genes associated with obesity making it a complex disease. And how our bodies function changes based on what we eat, when we eat, our weight and weight loss.

How our bodies adapt in response to weight loss makes maintaining weight loss difficult. The hormone ghrelin, which stimulates our appetite, increases when we lose weight and leptin, along with other gut hormones that suppress our appetite, decreases. A better understanding of these gut hormones that help regulate appetite has led to the discovery of medications, most available by prescription, that can help with appetite regulation. But they are still not magic pills that allow us to eat what we want, not exercise and still lose weight. Weight loss medications can help us lose weight, but we still must put in the work and make the changes.

"Health at any size" is a phrase you may have heard, so why lose weight? Research has shown that obese adults have a significantly increased risk of death from cardiovascular disease and a shorter life span. Carrying extra weight is also linked to an increased risk of Type 2 diabetes, osteoarthritis, fatty liver diseases, gall bladder problems, kidney disease, sleep apnea and fertility and pregnancy problems. And the big C – cancer. The studies are observational but according to the National Cancer Institute, the evidence consistently supports that being overweight or obese can increase the risk for endometrial, esophageal, stomach, kidney, liver, colon, pancreatic and other cancers. Researchers are still sorting out the whys, but the relationship between health and weight are there. Studies show that even a 7%-10% weight loss will reduce your risk of disease significantly.

Weight loss and maintaining weight loss involves permanently changing behaviors instead of short-term, quick fixes. Ask yourself before you begin a weight loss journey why you have decided to lose weight. Identify at least three reasons and why they are important to you and review them daily to reinforce your decision to make permanent lifestyle changes. Learning new habits will make it easier for you to reach and maintain your goals. Readiness is the key.

Weight gain comes easy. A 2010 study in the *Journal of the American Medical Association* found that most Americans gain about 1.5 pounds a year from age 25 to 55. For some, the gradual weight gain is because of metabolism, genetics, hormones, less activity and exercise, and an increase in calories. Even sleep habits play a role. The Sleep Medicine Program at the New York University School of Medicine suggests that the hormones leptin and ghrelin are affected by lack of sleep, which may affect our drive to eat. Lower levels of leptin mean we don't feel satisfied after eating and higher levels of ghrelin increases appetite.

Dr. Kevin Hall at the National Institute of Diabetes and Digestive and Kidney Diseases reports that by just adding 10 calories daily over thirty years you can gain as much as 20 pounds. In 2006, over 70% of Americans dieted. Yet studies have shown that most people do not maintain weight loss. While diets usually dictate what to eat, they don't consider food preferences, culture, schedule, or lifestyle.

One of the best studies is from the National Weight Control Registry, co-founded in 1994 by Rena Wing, professor of psychiatry and human behavior at Brown University. It is the largest ongoing study of people who lost weight and kept it off. The study follows about 6,000 individuals who had lost an average of 55 pounds and maintained the weight loss for at least 1 year. On average, participants have maintained the weight loss for 6 years. These individuals took a simple and practical approach by choosing behavior changes they could live with.

Losing and maintaining weight loss will require developing a good relationship with food and exercise. But it's not all or nothing. Small changes in calories and activity can result in weight loss that is permanent.

Characteristics of "Weight Losers"

- They used a combination of diet and exercise.
- About half worked with a dietitian or joined Weight Watchers. Women liked having help, while men tended to go it alone.
- Some counted calories; others counted fat grams.
- Many limited high calorie foods like desserts.

How Did They Keep it Off?

- Tracked their food intake.
- Ate breakfast regularly.
- Walked about an hour a day or burned the same calories with other activities.
- Watched TV fewer than 10 hours a week.
- Weighed themselves at least once a week.
- Followed regular meal plans and didn't splurge much on holidays and special occasions.
- Limited how often they ate out.
- They dined out an average of three times a week and ate fast foods less than once a week.

MEASURING WEIGHT AND PROGRESS

There are different ways to determine what you should weigh. Height and weight tables do not consider age, muscle mass, weight history, or genetics.

Waist circumference gages visceral fat, which is found deep in the abdomen around organs. Generally, men should have a waist no larger than 40 inches, and women no larger than 35 inches. An increase in 2 inches can raise the risk of metabolic syndrome by 17%. The larger the waist, the more likely someone is to have large amounts of visceral fat, which has been linked to insulin resistance, Type 2 diabetes, hypertension, and heart disease. Weight loss can shrink those fat cells. Using a tape measure, start at the top of the hip bone and bring it around, level with your navel. Measure your waist just after breathing out.

One of the most widely used methods is the Body Mass Index (BMI). BMI takes your height and weight into account. BMI is calculated by dividing a person's weight in kilograms by their height in meters squared. ($BMI=kg/m2$ or $lbs./in2 \times 703$). On the table, find your height in inches in the left-hand column. Move across the row to your weight. The number at the top of the column is your BMI. There are also calculators on line.

An "normal" BMI is between 18.5 and 24.9. When the BMI climbs past the normal range, the risk of disease increases. A BMI below 18.5 is considered underweight and brings its own health risks, especially for people 65 and over. There are limitations to the BMI calculation. For muscular athletes, BMI may overestimate body fat. For the elderly or others who have depleted muscle mass, BMI may underestimate the body fat. BMI is an imperfect tool, but just one tool, used in determining and managing a healthy weight.

METABOLIC SYNDROME

A group of conditions increase the risk of heart disease, strokes, diabetes and other diseases. Three or more of the following are needed to be diagnosed with metabolic syndrome:

- Waist circumference of over 35 inches for women and over 40 inches for men.
- Triglycerides over 150.
- HDL less than 40 for men and less than 50 for women.
- Blood pressure greater 130/85 (either number).
- Fasting blood sugar over 100

DETERMINING BODY MASS INDEX (BMI)

BMI (Kg/m^2)	19	20	21	22	23	24	25	26	27	28	29	30	35	40
Height (in.)							Weight (lb.)							
58	91	96	100	105	110	115	119	124	129	134	138	143	167	191
59	94	99	104	109	114	119	124	128	133	138	143	148	173	198
60	97	102	107	112	118	123	128	133	138	143	148	153	179	204
61	100	106	111	116	122	127	132	137	143	148	153	158	185	211
62	104	109	115	120	126	131	136	142	147	153	158	164	191	218
63	107	113	118	124	130	135	141	146	152	158	163	169	197	225
64	110	116	122	128	134	140	145	151	157	163	169	174	204	232
65	114	120	126	132	138	144	150	156	162	168	174	180	210	240
66	118	124	130	136	142	148	155	161	167	173	179	186	216	247
67	121	127	134	140	146	153	159	166	172	178	185	191	223	255
68	125	131	138	144	151	158	164	171	177	184	190	197	230	262
69	128	135	142	149	155	162	169	176	182	189	196	203	236	270
70	132	139	146	153	160	167	174	181	188	195	202	207	243	278

71	136	143	150	157	165	172	179	186	193	200	208	215	250	286
72	140	147	154	162	169	177	184	191	199	206	213	221	258	294
73	144	151	159	166	174	182	189	197	204	212	219	227	265	302
74	148	155	163	171	179	186	194	202	210	218	225	233	272	311
75	152	160	168	176	184	192	200	208	216	224	232	240	279	319
76	156	164	172	180	189	197	205	213	221	230	238	246	287	328

Source: National Heart Lung & Blood Institute

BMI	Weight Category	Risk of disease
18.5 or less	Underweight	Low
18.5 - 24.9	Normal	Low
25.0 - 29.9	Overweight	High
30.0 - 34.9	Obese	Very High
35.0 - 39.9	Obese	Very High
40 or greater	Morbid Obese	Extremely High

HOW MUCH TO EAT?

We are all different when it comes to how many calories we need. Age, gender, physical activity, and metabolism all play a role. Men need more calories than women due to larger size and muscle mass. As we age, our calorie needs decrease due to a slower metabolism. It's important to match your energy intake (calories) with energy expenditure (physical activity) to avoid gaining weight

Studies have shown that most people underestimate their calorie intake by as much as 25%. For weight loss, reduce calories by 250-500 a day. Once you've reached your weight goal, your calorie needs may not be much more than what you were eating to lose weight. Regardless of age or gender, if you are very active, your calorie needs will be higher to maintain weight than those who are not active. Most moderately active women will lose weight consuming about 1200 to 1500 calories, men about 1800 to 2,000 calories.

Spend thirty minutes exercising and you'll burn about 200 calories. Choosemyplate.gov provides a calorie calculator based upon your age, weight, and activity level.

THE SCALE: FRIEND OR FOE

Weighing regularly can enhance your weight loss efforts. The scale provides immediate feedback. You'll see changes in your weight and can adjust your calories immediately. Keep in mind that pounds can come and go possibly due to fluid, exercise, sodium intake, or hormonal changes. By checking your weight at least once or twice a week you can determine if the number of calories you're eating are providing consistent weight loss of 3 to 8 pounds per month. Also, if you are always hungry and find yourself obsessing about food, you've probably reduced your calories too much. A steady weight loss of 1-2 pounds per month provides the opportunity to make permanent behavior changes. Once you reach your weight goal, the scale can keep you on track. If you find yourself up a few pounds you can quickly assess your eating and exercise and adjust.

PUT FOOD IN WRITING

A food log helps keep you honest with yourself. Studies show that people who track their calories lose twice as much weight as those who don't.

TOP PHONE APPS

The top apps for weight management from Sarah Krieger MPH, RD, LDN and the Academy of Nutrition and Dietetics (eatright.org)

Calorie Counter: Tracks food, exercise, weight and the nutrients listed on a nutrition label. Includes inspirational articles, healthy recipes, and a help section. Rating: 4 stars

Calorie Counter & Diet Tracker by MyFitnessPal: Tracks fitness goals and nutrients. Rating: 4.5 stars

Calorie Counter: Diets & Activities: Features a food diary that tracks calories, water, fitness and the time each food item is eaten, and body tracker. An option allows you to create your own diet and physical activity. Rating: 4 stars

Calorie Tracker by Livestrong.com: Food and fitness diary. Rating: 4 stars

Lose it: Keeps track of foods you eat with a detailed food database. Primarily for people who want to lose weight. Rating: 3 stars

Sparkpeople Food and Fitness Tracker: Fitness and food tracker for people looking to lose a ½ pound to 2 pounds per week or to maintain weight. Rating: 4 stars

FOOD LOG TIPS

Write down everything you eat and drink, no matter how small. Food diary apps are helpful.

1. Write down how much you ate, and the calories if available. Write it down as soon after eating as possible.
2. Write how you felt before, during, and after eating.
3. Record your physical activity.
4. Total the calories after each meal so you know how much you have left in your daily budget.
5. Record your weight once or twice a week so you see the relationship between calories eaten and your weight.
6. Write down everything you eat and drink, no matter how small. Food diary apps are helpful.
7. Write down how much you ate, and the calories if available.

Food logs should include food, portions, calories, time, place, activity, and feelings. It's worth the effort. You'll identify why and what you eat. You can create an environment that makes it easier to be successful.

Food logs help identify unnecessary eating allowing you to reconsider whether you want to spend your calories on a particular food.

Make sure your food log is portable and keep it within reach. With today's technology, some individuals keep their calories logged on smartphones, tablets, or laptop computers. Free apps such as Lose It and My Fitness Pal make calorie counting easy. The book *Calorie King* can be used or the website www.calorieking.com. The book *Bite It & Write It: A Guide to Keeping Track of What You Eat & Drink* is another food journal available.

SETTING UP FOR SUCCESS

- Don't buy high calorie foods.
- Buy lower-calorie snacks you enjoy.
- Store tempting foods out of sight.
- Avoid buffets when eating out.
- Put fresh fruit on the counter or table rather than in the refrigerator.
- Portion snacks ahead of time.
- Take your own healthy snacks to work or when running errands.
- Use smaller plates, bowls, and glasses.
- Read labels for calorie information.
- Include small portions of your favorite foods occasionally; it is the frequency and quantity that counts.

FINDING BALANCE

Think of your calorie quota like a budget. You have a certain amount to "spend" each day, and like any budget, you must adjust your expenditures to stay within that limit. By counting calories no foods are forbidden, and you can adjust calories to include foods and beverages you might otherwise avoid. Newer research gives us insight into the differences in foods and the energy needed to digest and process the food. One study showed that people who received 25% of their calories from protein burned 227 calories a day more than those who only ate 5% of their calories from protein. Another study found that people who ate whole grains vs. refined grains burned about 100 calories more a day. So smart calorie counting means including your favorite foods occasionally but emphasizes a balanced diet of mostly nutrient-dense lean protein, whole grains, vegetables and fruits and fewer refined carbohydrates, less saturated fats, and less added sugar. You'll eliminate the guilt that comes with eating high calorie items and improve your relationship with food.

Subtotal calories after meals and snacks so you have a running account of how many calories you've spent and what you have left. If you find yourself eating more at lunch than you had planned, you can balance your calorie budget by eating less at dinner. Avoid the mindset that if a food is "good for you" it doesn't count. All foods have calories, so they all matter. Even excessive amounts of fruits or beverages can interfere with losing weight.

CHARACTERISTICS OF OVERWEIGHT INDIVIDUALS

- They eat the most of their calories in the evening.
- They skip breakfast and sometimes lunch.
- They snack after dinner.

Recording what you eat helps identify eating patterns and emotions that can lead to grazing and mindless eating. It can also serve as a reminder to eat! People who skip meals may shift most of their calories to the evening and overeat. The result: Grabbing fast foods and not much time left to burn off those calories!

REMEMBER

"Eat breakfast like a king, lunch like a prince, and dinner like a pauper."

Life can interfere with plans. Work days and commutes are longer, our children have more activities, and dinner is often later. But a study in the *Journal of Human Nutrition and Dietetics* found that those who ate most of their calories in the evening were two times more likely to be overweight than those who ate more of their calories in the early or mid-day

EMOTIONAL EATING

By writing how you feel when you eat (happy, stressed, tired) you will also connect your mood and what, when, why, and how much you eat. This understanding will allow you to work out behaviors that cause you to eat less healthy foods and overeat. We use food as comfort when under stress, bored, anxious, or sad. The temporary feel good that comes with high calorie foods is a quick fix. Using your food log, you can name those emotions, recognize triggers, and begin to work on managing them more constructively. You can learn to short circuit an impulse to eat during those emotional moments and substitute different methods to process and handle stress and other powerful emotions. Use an activity that matches that feeling or mood. If you're tired, take a nap. If stressed or worried, distract yourself by doing yoga or taking a walk. If you're struggling to manage on your own, then it may be time to seek more support and help working through issues.

THE FULLNESS FACTOR AND SNACKS

Individual foods have what we refer to as a satiety index, or "fullness factor." Satiety is the power of food we've eaten to decrease our desire to eat more. Foods with high satiety power or fullness factor are thought to help control how much we eat and as a result, our weight. Foods with protein, fiber, fat and water keep you feeling full longer and more satisfied. So, if you find yourself hungry in the middle of the afternoon, choose a snack that will prevent you from being ravenous by dinnertime.

Most women should keep snacks around 100 to 150 calories, men 150 to 200 calories. Choose snacks that you enjoy within that calorie level. Determine your satiety index by tracking when you get hungry after eating those snacks.

If dinner is pushed late into the evening, try appetizers or splitting a meal rather than eating a large meal late at night. Shift more of your calories earlier in the day to avoid being hungry.

A good rule is: The later the dinner, the fewer the calories. Plan and you can keep your calorie budget balance.

HIGH SATIETY SNACKS

- 1 slice cheese
- 15 almonds
- Large apple
- ½ cup cottage cheese
- No-fat yogurt
- 1 oz. chocolate
- 3 cups popcorn

DON'T SKIP MEALS TO LOSE WEIGHT

- Make breakfast a priority. Whether running to make an appointment, dropping kids off at school, or catching a plane. Take time to eat or drink something nutritious. Include at least 7 grams of protein.

Planning is the key.

Break for lunch. Eat a lunch with at least 300 calories. Pack a lunch if you're on the run. It takes only a few extra minutes in the morning or the night before to pull together a nutritious meal. If you spend a lot of time in the car, keep a cooler packed with water, fruit, cheese, and other portable foods. If eating out, use calories listed on menus, menu boards or online to help you stay within your calorie budget. If you eat lunch out, try to eat dinner at home. Or, if your schedule includes dinner out, try to pack a lunch.

- Plan for dinner. Think ahead to dinner and plan for the calories. Have foods available that can be quickly prepared. There are many cookbooks with 30 minute or less recipes. Try the Easy Meal chapter.
- Watch your portions.

WEIGHT GAIN AND MENOPAUSE

The weight gain that accompanies menopause can be frustrating and seems to sneak up on most women. Hormones are in a state of flux—estrogen declines, and testosterone increases—influencing the distribution of fat. During this time women can gain as much as 15 pounds, and most weight settles in the middle, leaving most women wondering what happened to their waist. Body shape changes and fat shifts from arms, legs, and hips to the abdomen. Visceral fat also increases during menopause.

Be proactive. Metabolism decreases during menopause, so women need to review and adjust their calorie intake if gaining weight. You may need to decrease your daily calories by 200 to 300 calories or increase your activity. Weighing regularly (at least weekly) can prevent weight from sneaking up on you. Many adults decrease their protein intake as they age just when it is becoming even more important, especially the amino acid leucine. According to researcher Christos Katsanos at Arizona State University, more amino acids are needed to stimulate protein synthesis (building new muscle). Animal protein (meat, poultry, dairy, fish, and eggs) are the best sources. Whey also contains leucine. He suggests aiming for at least 20 grams of protein at each meal. Others recommend 30 grams of protein at each meal. Spread the protein over the course of the day and eat a source of protein after a workout. The U.S. dietary guidelines recommend 0.8 grams of protein (or more) for every 2.2 pounds of body weight. For example, a person who weighs 150 pounds should take in about 56 grams of protein a day. A 4-ounce chicken breast has about 28 grams, a glass of milk 8 grams and 5 ounces Greek yogurt about 13 grams.

Stay active. Increasing activity is just as important as reducing calories to avoid weight gain. We begin losing about a quarter pound of muscle each year beginning in our late 30s or early 40s. More muscle means burning more calories. Women who exercise at least 30 minutes daily gain the least amount of weight. The *Journal of the American Medical Association* reports that women need 60 minutes of moderate-intensity exercise daily to avoid weight gain as they move from their twenties and thirties into middle age. Researchers from the University of Pittsburg also found that individuals avoided weight gain by following a diet of 1300 calories and by doing exercise that burns 150 to 200 calories per day. Weight strengthening exercises build muscle, slow muscle loss, and increase bone density. Researcher James E. Grave, dean of the College of Health at the University of Utah found older adults who maintain muscle mass can avoid some health problems including disability and loss of independence. In a separate study Dr. Mark D. Peterson found that adults between ages 50 and 90 gained an average of nearly 2.5 pounds of lean body mass primarily muscle with about 20 weeks of resistance training with weights and exercise. Start early and start slow, gradually increasing the intensity and frequency of workouts. This is especially important for the menopausal woman whose body is undergoing so many changes. A combination of aerobic and weight strengthening is best. Visit with a registered dietitian and a personal trainer to develop a program that's just right for you.

No matter what your age, losing, and maintaining weight is a complicated process and requires vigilance. A study published in *American Journal of Clinical Nutrition* found that women, (average age 58) who lost 25 pounds and regained weight, the pounds returned as fat mass rather than muscle mass.

AVOIDING WEIGHT GAIN

- Know the calories you require to lose or maintain weight
- Eat a consistent diet most days
- Don't skip meals
- Stay active. Exercise at least 30 minutes a day
- Weigh yourself regularly
- Avoid allowing a small weight gain to turn into more

FAD DIETS: SUDDEN, QUICK-SPREADING, AND SHORT-LIVED

Weight loss claims that seem too good to be true. That's one thing that fad diets have in common. Fad diets have been around for decades. Most individuals stick with the diet for a few months and then return to their old eating style and the pounds creep back. But weight loss isn't just about losing weight, it's about *maintaining* that weight loss

Weight maintenance programs have shown that individuals who aren't deprived of favorite high-calorie foods, but instead watch portion sizes, have a better success rate at losing and maintaining weight loss. These participants successfully maintained their weight loss because they did not view their dietary changes as temporary. They made lifestyle changes.

Fad diets can be risky for individuals with certain health conditions. Fad diets have also been found to place individuals at risk of coronary disease, cancer, gout, kidney stones, osteoporosis, keto-breath, fainting, dizziness, and high blood pressure.

Some new diets have entered the fad diet scene, for better or worse. Below are some of the new diets and what they are about. As always, diet at your own risk, we recommended making sustainable lifestyle changes.

Paleo Diet

- High in protein
- Low to moderate carbohydrate
- Low in sodium and refined sugar
- Restricts high glycemic foods
- Restricts dairy foods

Glycemic Index Diet

- Generally, restricts high calorie foods such as desserts, breads, and pastas. These can cause rapid blood sugar rise, insulin secretion, and possible weight gain.
- Following a glycemic index diet can lead to weight loss because higher caloric foods are discouraged. However, it eliminates some lower calorie nutrient rich foods.
- Watching glycemic index does not help individuals to learn how to eat healthfully and does not encourage exercise as part of the plan.

Detox Diet

- A short-term diet
- Often cuts out entire foods groups or is limited to liquids
- Encourages organic foods
- Risks include nutritional deficiencies
- Headaches
- Diarrhea leading to dehydration and electrolyte loss
- Constipation if not drinking enough water with increased fiber
- Fatigue

- Not appropriate for most, but especially pregnant or nursing mothers, children, individuals with eating disorders, those with chronic diseases such as diabetes, thyroid disease, or kidney disease

Intermittent Fasting

- This involves limiting food intake two days a week to 500 calories daily. Food is eaten in an eight-hour window, typically 10 am-6 pm. Other types include fasting for 24 hours one to two days a week, or consuming foods only within an eight-hour window.
- Risks include fatigue
- Inadequate carbohydrate on fasting days can limit healthy exercise
- Fasting can lead to overeating during non-fast times
- Individuals who should not follow the diet include all the above under detox diets

As dietitians, we have seen there is no BEST diet for weight loss. Short term high protein, low carbohydrate diets may provide a jump-start, but requires caution to prevent harmful results. We feel that the Mediterranean diet with its high quality foods is an effective dietary plan supported by many.

It is important to focus on following a diet with negative energy balance, and quality foods to promote good health. Long-term success will be assured with adherence.

EXERCISE: KEY TO FITNESS, HEALTH, AND HAPPINESS

"We are under exercised as a nation. We look, instead of play. We ride, instead of walk. Our existence deprives us of the minimum of physical activity essential for healthy living."

— *Former President John F. Kennedy*

xercise Questions: Test your knowledge by answering True or False to the questions below.

1. Schedule conflicts and time constraints can keep people from exercising regularly

2. To reduce the risk of chronic disease, Americans should aim for at least 30 minutes of physical activity 3-5 times per week

3. Health clubs are a great place for everyone, especially busy people, to exercise

4. If you schedule exercise, you are more likely to exercise

5. Activity and exercise can have a significant impact on weight

6. Excluding exercise from a weight loss plan is okay

7. Planning ways to incorporate exercise into the day shows a willingness to make change.

8. Working mothers have no time to exercise and cannot increase their activity level.

GETTING STARTED AND MAKING IT WORK

The Physical Activity Guidelines for Americans, released by the U.S. Department of Health and Human Services, recommends that adults get at least 150 minutes of moderate-intensity physical activity a week and perform muscle-strengthening exercises two or more days each week.

Advanced technology, long days at work, and sitting at computers all day can affect our health and weight. But just moving makes a difference. Researchers at Mayo Clinic studied a small group of people who consumed more calories than their body burned for two months. They tracked their fat storage and the number of calories burned during normal activity. Those who moved more gained less fat than those that did not. All those extra steps matter – taking the stairs, parking farther away – add up, so look for opportunities to move around during the day. Take phone calls standing up or pace as you talk. Stand, stretch, bend; anything is better than sitting still. But a regular exercise routine is even better. It creates a habit that supports physical and mental health, strength, stamina, and flexibility that will pay off. Exercise is an investment in you and your long-term health and well-being as you age

Studies show that the frailty that comes with age can be reduced significantly through exercise. Dr. Cheryl Phillips, president of the American Geriatric Society states, "Physical activity is more powerful than any medication a senior can take."

10 REASONS TO EXERCISE:

1. Helps maintain weight
2. Promotes healthy bones
3. Helps lose weight
4. Increases muscle mass
5. Improves blood circulation

6. Reduces stress

7. Improves blood pressure

8. Decreases risk for diabetes and other chronic diseases

9. Improves mood

10. May allow you to eat more

SELECTING AN EXERCISE

Exercise, like a pair of shoes, must be a good fit to work. If you are just starting to exercise, start with activities that are not too intense, such as walking or biking. Outdoor activities such as walking, running, or biking are great when the weather is warm, but when the temperature drops, so often does the exercise routine. If you decide on an outdoor activity, have a back-up plan for bad weather days. Invest in indoor exercise equipment if possible, such as a treadmill or stationary bike. Treadmills allow you to walk and run and control the intensity of your workout with speed and incline.

Some people prefer the structure and comradery of exercise classes. Spinning and dance classes are fun indoor activities. Some studies show that those that participate in group classes tend to stick with the program longer than those who exercise alone. Most important is to choose an exercise that is enjoyable and sustainable. Being flexible with the type of exercise, time and place increases the odds that you'll stick with it.

Check with your doctor before exercising if:

- You have cardiovascular disease
- You have musculoskeletal problems
- You have neurological abnormalities
- You have cardiac, pulmonary, or metabolic diseases -you should begin your exercise in a medically supervised environment

If you can't afford equipment or don't have the room, take advantage of exercise programs on television, online or DVD.

TIPS FOR SCHEDULING EXERCISE

- Measure your activity with a pedometer(a device you wear that counts your steps throughout the day) and translates into miles or kilometers.
- Keep exercise clothes with you in the car so you can stop at the gym whenever you have time.
- Find opportunities to exercise if you find yourself waiting for an appointment or a child at an activity.
- When traveling, try to find hotels that have a fitness room or pool.
- Partner with a colleague or friend and exercise together.
- Bypass the elevator and use the stairs when possible.
- Avoid planning exercises that are too time-consuming for your schedule.

PERSONAL TRAINERS

If you decide a personal trainer is right for you, find one that is certified and experienced. Certification should come from a well-known organization such as the Cooper Institute, the National Academy of Sports Medicine, the American College of Sports Medicine, the American Council on Exercise, or the National Strength and Conditioning Association. You can also look for a certified trainer online at www.ideafit.com or the ACSM website at www.acsm.org. Before choosing a trainer, observe them working with other clients or ask friends for a referral. Some trainers may offer a free trial session

A trainer can help evaluate your body composition as well as put together a program that includes cardiovascular fitness, flexibility, and strength training. If you have a history of medical complications such as heart attacks, diabetes, or injuries, talk to your doctor before starting any exercise program. Your doctor may want to refer you to a physical therapist who will be able to incorporate all your medical issues into an exercise program designed for you.

HEALTH CLUBS

Pros

Easy to find

Variety of equipment

Group classes such as yoga, weight training, kickboxing, spinning, and dance

Personal trainers

Socializing

Multiple locations – many have locations across the country for traveling

Cons

Price

Travel time to and from a health club

Waiting for machines during peak times

Time exercising before or after work requires extra time for a shower and change of clothes.

TIPS FOR SETTING FITNESS GOALS

Start your exercise program by establishing fitness goals and developing a plan to achieve them.

1. **Evaluate your current level of activity.** You may be surprised at how much you move throughout the day. A pedometer or app on your phone is an easy way to provide an initial assessment of your activity level. After wearing a pedometer for a day or two, you can then set a goal to increase your activity. A goal for most individuals is 10,000 steps daily, which roughly equals 5 miles. The average person walks about 2-3 miles per day doing daily activities. Listed below is a chart with step goals per day.

2. **Set short-term goals first,** such as biking for 20 minutes three times a week. Achieving short-term goals will provide motivation to continue with a program.

3. **Start Slowly.** It's not all or nothing. If you miss a workout, just pick up where you left off. It's important to stay positive and be encouraging to yourself, just as you would be to others.

4. **Include strength-training.** Strength training should be done at least 2-3 times per week. It can prevent age-related loss of muscle mass and bone density. It can also help you move better. Choose moves that focus on big muscle groups like the legs, butt, and back such as lunges, squats, and rows.

5. **Exercise in short blocks throughout the day.** Your exercise does not have to be all at one time. Instead of trying to block off a 30-minute chunk of time, two 15-minute chunks may fit your schedule better three times a week. Achieving short-term goals will provide motivation to continue with a program.

6. **It's not all or nothing.** If you miss a workout, just pick up where you left off. It's important to stay positive and be encouraging to yourself, just as you would be to others.

Steps per day	Miles walked per day	Level of activity
2,000	1.0	Low
5,000	2.5	Medium
10,000	5.0	Optimal

TARGET HEART RATE

You get the most out of your workout when your heart rate is at a target rate that is right for your age and health. At your target heart rate, you are burning fat at the highest pace for your body. To find your target heart rate, you need to first find your maximum heart rate. This is calculated at 220 minus your age. Your target heart rate is between 50% and 75% of your maximum heart rate. You can also use the table listed below. It is recommended when beginning an exercise program to aim for the lower end of your target heart rate and gradually increase.

Age	Target heart rate zone (50%-75%) beats per minute	Average maximum heart rate (100%) beats per minute
20	100 - 150	200
25	98 - 146	195
30	94 - 142	190
35	93 - 138	185
40	90 - 135	180
45	88 - 131	175
50	85 - 127	170
55	83 - 123	165
60	80 - 120	160
65	78 - 116	155
70	75 - 113	150

HURRY UP AND ... WAIT

Do you ever find yourself rushing somewhere only to find that you must sit and wait? Take that time back and get moving with these tips.

- Keep a pair of good walking shoes with you, in your desk or car, for unplanned exercise. Measure the distance you've walked and the calories burned.

- If you arrive somewhere early, go for a walk. Waiting for your kid's baseball game to end? Athletic fields often have a walking path surrounding them. In office buildings, walk the hallways and up and down stairs. Stairs can give you a workout that becomes cardiovascular if done for several minutes.

- If several of your appointments are in the same area, park the car and walk to each one. Park as far away as you can from an appointment to force yourself to walk further.

- Stuck waiting in the airport? Put away the phone, tablet and laptop and get some walking done. Skip the moving walkways. Those extra minutes add up.

MAINTAINING AN EXERCISE PROGRAM

- **List reasons for exercise**. Put the list in a place you will see it every day, like the bathroom mirror, refrigerator, your desk, or your car's dashboard. This will help reinforce exercise.

- **Find your motivation by asking a friend.** Ask people who exercise regularly why they do so. Find out what motivates them and how they work around his own schedule conflicts. Many busy people find ways to never miss their exercise.

- **Make exercise a routine.** Exercise is like taking a shower or brushing your teeth. The more you resist the temptation not to exercise, the less you'll feel that temptation and exercise will become a part of your day.

- **Vary your exercise routine.** Try a new exercise before you have the chance to get bored with what you are doing.

Discover winter. Winter can be a great time to exercise outdoors if you dress appropriately. Clear cold days and nights are perfect for a brisk walk or run. Take the dog or borrow a neighbor's. Better yet, volunteer at a shelter to walk dogs. You'll soon have a new buddy or two. Each season of the year has advantages, and seeing the different seasons on foot can be rewarding.

- **Vary exercise times.** Remember that exercise does not have to be done all at once. Try doing 15 minutes in the morning and another 15 minutes in the evening if that's what best fits your schedule.
- **Exercise with a friend.** This can be more fun and motivating. When you are both committed to a plan together, you can motivate each other and are less likely to skip a workout.

IT'S A DATE

Write your exercise schedule in your planner or add to your phone/ computer calendar at the beginning of each week. Make a date with yourself. However, be flexible if something forces you to miss your exercise date. Immediately reschedule any missed exercise to better stay on track.

CHART YOUR PROGRESS

An excellent way to keep up your motivation is to keep an exercise log. Record your workout goals and how you want to achieve them. Then record what you accomplished at each workout and the time you spent.

A log can help track your progress and allow adjustments to your exercise routine as needed. As with a food log, an exercise log will hold you accountable for your fitness goals and keep you on track. It may also help you to identify situations that interfere with your goals and tell you when it is time to set higher goals.

FUELING FOR PERFORMANCE

For those that are already regularly exercising or training for an event, staying hydrated and fueled is crucial. Carbohydrates fuel your muscles and brain. Dehydration (fluid loss) and hyponatremia (sodium loss) should also be a big concern. During training, find meals, snacks, and fluids that work best for you. Have your own personal recipe for fueling for success.

- Sweat contains electrolytes that keep the fluid inside and outside your cells in balance.

- Know your sweat rate. Begin by identifying your hourly fluid loss (especially when training for events) by weighing nude before and after a run and before eating and drinking. Any weight loss represents fluid loss, and you can base fluid needs on this. A 2% loss in weight represents dehydration, and you can lose your ability to perform well. A 9% to 12% loss can cause death.

- Check your urine. Light-colored urine means you're well hydrated. Dark colored urine may indicate you need more fluids.

- Drink before you feel thirsty. Besides water, sweat contains electrolytes that keep the fluid inside and outside of your cells in balance.

- Drink water throughout the day. Before a run of 2 hours or more, drink about 10 to 24 ounces and an additional 8 ounces 10 to 20 minutes before the run. Eat a few salty snacks to stimulate your thirst and help retain fluid.

- Avoid over hydrating. Drinking too much can lead to a dilution of your blood sodium resulting in hyponatremia.

- Choose sports drinks that contain 14 to 19 grams of carbohydrate per 8 ounces. Higher concentrations of carbs can upset the stomach. They also contain sodium and potassium that can be lost through sweat.

- Replace fluid loss with 16 to 24 ounces of fluid for every pound of weight loss. If you become dehydrated, drink frequently for the next day or two.

- Eat high carbohydrate meals daily to fuel your muscles while training. The night before an event, eat a high carbohydrate meal and drink extra fluids.

- Start the day of an event with a combination of carbohydrates such as a bagel and banana and protein such as cheese or peanut butter.

- Soon after an event, for optimal recovery, eat carbohydrates and protein. Include 1-1.2 grams of carbohydrate per kilogram (2.2 lbs.) of body weight to replenish glycogen stores. Consume 20-25 grams of protein for muscle recovery. Dairy products are good choices because they contain carbohydrates and protein as well as sodium and potassium.

EXERCISE AND STRONGER BONES

Muscle mass loss can begin as early as our 30s and 40s. The rate is even higher for individuals in their 60s; the average bone loss is around 3% per year. The August 2012 *Journal of the American Academy of Nutrition and Dietetics* suggests that people age 60 and older increase their protein intake. Foods rich in the amino acid leucine seem to stimulate muscle protein synthesis. Try for 25 to 30 grams of protein at each meal. Good sources include lean meat, poultry, fish, eggs, dairy products, lentils and beans, soy foods and nuts.

Getting adequate calcium and vitamin D are crucial to building strong bones. Numerous studies have found, however, that there is as strong a relationship between exercise and improvement in bone mineral density. These studies have shown that the pull of muscle on bone stimulates bone growth and allows bone to become stronger and denser. High impact exercise allows muscles and bones to work against gravity to build strength. Combining resistance and strength-training exercise helps to not only build bone but also builds muscle that supports the skeleton and improves balance and posture. Greater bone health stronger muscles can help prevent falls that lead to fractures. Dr. Miriam Nelson, director of Tufts University's John Hancock Research on Physical Activity, Nutrition, and Obesity Prevention recommends an exercise program that combines aerobic, weight, and strength training.

High Impact Exercise

- Dancing
- High Impact Aerobics
- Hiking
- Jogging or Running
- Jumping Rope
- Racquetball
- Tennis
- Volleyball

Low Impact Exercise

- Elliptical Training machine use
- Fast walking, treadmill or outdoors
- Stair-step machine
- Low impact aerobics

Non-weight bearing Exercise

- Bicycling
- Indoor Cycling
- Deep water walking
- Flexibility exercise
- Stretching exercises
- Swimming
- Water aerobics

Answers to Exercise Questions:

1. True
2. False - Americans should exercise for at least 30 minutes daily.
3. False - Getting to and from a health club and waiting to use equipment may take extra time.
4. True
5. True
6. False - Skipping exercise will make it more difficult to lose weight.
7. True
8. False - Carefully looking at your schedule will allow you to find ways to incorporate exercise.

MINDFUL EATING

Mindful Eating is a technique that is being used by many dietitians to help individuals gain control over eating habits. It helps treat emotional eating triggers and external eating that occurs in response to the sight or smell of food.

Mindful eating teaches you skills to deal with eating impulses. It places you in control of your food responses rather than allowing you to succumb to your food instincts.

Mindful Eating has 6 categories:

1. Observe

   Notice your body. Rumbling stomach, low energy, stressed out, satisfied, full, empty etc.

2. In-the Moment

   Being fully present. Turn off the television, put away your book or newspaper. Sit down. Focus on eating and nothing else. Stop multitasking. Designate a spot just for eating and no other activities.

3. Savor

   Notice the texture, aroma, and flavor of your food. Is it crunchy, sweet, salty, smooth, or spicy?

4. Nonjudgment

   Speak mindfully and compassionately. Notice when "should", rigid rules or guilt pop into your mind.

5. Awareness

   Tasting your food versus mindless eating. Take your time and slow down your eating.

6. Make your eating atmosphere pleasant. Use dishes and utensils you enjoy. If you come home stressed or upset, allow yourself some time to decompress and feel better before eating.

Use your 5 senses to increase your enjoyment and satisfaction of your food. This contributes to a sensual, satisfying food experience.

SIGHT

- Pick a pleasant eating environment
- Eat on an attractive eating surface
- Choose utensils, plates etc. that you enjoy
- Place your food attractively on the plate

SOUND

- Listen to the sound of cooking
- Be aware of conversation
- Avoid unpleasant discussions during mealtimes
- Listen to pleasant background music

SMELL

- Pay attention to the smell of food while being cooked and before you eat
- Appreciate the smell of the seasonings and the food once it is on the plate

FEEL

- Touch the texture of the table where the food is served
- Detect the feeling of the utensils, napkins, and plates
- Be aware of the textures of the food
- Notice the temperature of the foods

TASTE

- Chew your food thoughtfully
- Analyze the flavors of the food
- Eat your food slowly and be aware of the food served
- Try one food at a time and appreciate the flavors of each food

SECTION 3

DIGGING IN ON NUTRITION

CHOLESTEROL & FAT: GET TO THE HEART OF THE MATTER

"He who takes medicine and neglects to diet wastes the skill of his doctors."

— *Chinese Proverb*

Cholesterol Questions: Test your knowledge by answering True or False.

1. I should have my cholesterol checked yearly by my doctor.
2. My desirable total cholesterol should be less than 200 mg/dL.
3. There is no difference between HDL cholesterol and LDL cholesterol; they should both be low.
4. To lower my cholesterol, I only have to lower my dietary cholesterol intake.
5. The main source of dietary cholesterol is fruits and vegetables.
6. Most cholesterol in the body comes from the pancreas.
7. Palm oil and coconut oil are high in saturated fat.

When we think of cholesterol and fat, we often think of heart disease. Heart disease remains the leading cause of death for men and women in the U.S. Approximately half of adults have some form of heart disease, and more than 80% of heart disease is said to be preventable. The 2019 Cardiovascular Disease Prevention Guidelines says that the best way to prevent cardiovascular disease is a healthy lifestyle that includes regular physical activity and healthy eating across the lifespan. A plant-based diet that includes vegetables, fruits, whole grains, nuts, lean protein and monounsaturated fats remains the healthiest eating style. The Mediterranean Diet is perhaps one of the best examples of a healthy diet. In the Mediterranean eating pattern, plant-based protein is provided by whole grains, lentils, legumes and beans, nuts and seeds.

But cholesterol and saturated fat remain one of the most controversial topics in the medical profession. More recent studies show that eating foods that naturally contain cholesterol don't increase blood cholesterol levels as once thought. Research has found that people who received most of their protein from meat had a 60% increase risk of cardiovascular disease versus a 40% risk for people whose protein source was mostly from nuts and seeds.

The 2020-2025 U.S. Dietary Guidelines contain some revision and yet many recommendations remain the same. For those 2 years and older saturated fat should be limited to less than 10 percent of calories per day. These fats can be replaced with unsaturated fats particularly polyunsaturated. The guidelines also recommend shifting to a plant-based diet by increasing intake of seafood, legumes, dairy products, whole grains, vegetables, fruits and a decrease in meats, sugar-sweetened foods and drinks, and refined grains.

IN THE KNOW: WHAT IS CHOLESTEROL?

Cholesterol is a soft fat-like substance that makes up part of our cells and tissues. During digestion of fat, cholesterol and fats are packaged together as lipoproteins, which allows cholesterol to travel through the body. The liver makes some cholesterol, but the remainder of the cholesterol in our bodies comes from food, mostly animal products. All animals naturally produce cholesterol; animal fat and skin are the main sources of cholesterol in the diet

4 TYPES OF LIPOPROTEINS ON YOUR LAB REPORT

- **Very low-density lipoprotein (VLDL) cholesterol.** VLDL carries fats to different parts of the body. VLDL is made in the liver and helps make LDL cholesterol.

- **Low-density lipoprotein (LDL) cholesterol.** LDL carries cholesterol to different parts of the body, and it is considered the "bad" cholesterol because it can stick to the inside of our blood vessels, making it harder for blood to pass through. This may increase our risk of heart disease. The size and density of LDL cholesterol are important. Large buoyant particles are associated with heart health while small dense particles are associated with a higher risk for heart disease.

- Weight loss and reducing refined carbohydrates may reduce small dense particles.

- **High-density lipoprotein (HDL) cholesterol.** This is known as the "good" cholesterol because HDL carries cholesterol away from blood vessel walls and back to the liver. The liver breaks down cholesterol to be excreted or recycled into new VLDL. Having more HDL and less LDL is beneficial.

- **Triglycerides.** Triglycerides are found in food and body fat. Your body stores extra calories as triglycerides. Having a high triglyceride level is often associated with a low HDL level, which is associated with an increased risk of heart disease. To lower triglycerides, reduce intake of refined carbohydrates and alcohol and increase physical activity.

One of the goals in managing cardiovascular disease is raising HDL cholesterol since HDL protects against heart disease. The National Cholesterol Education Program Adult Treatment Panel III recommends lifestyle changes as first-line treatment for increasing HDL cholesterol if levels are below 40 mg/dL for men and below 50 for women. Exercise of moderate intensity more than three times per week will increase HDL cholesterol an average of 4%. A decrease of 1kg (2.2 lbs.) of body weight in overweight adults will increase HDL cholesterol by an average of 1%. Stopping smoking may lead to a 3% to 5.6% increase in HDL cholesterol levels.

MORE ABOUT CHOLESTEROL

Heart Disease

Major factors for heart disease include:

- Family history of heart disease
- Being 45 years or older for men or 55 years or older for a woman
- Smoking
- High blood pressure
- Diabetes

Target levels for blood lipids	
Total Cholesterol	less than 200 mg/dL
LDL Cholesterol	less than 100 mg/dL
HDL Cholesterol	at least 40 mg/dL for men at least 50 mg/dL for women
Triglycerides	less than 150 mg/dL
Total Cholesterol: HDL Ratio	less than 3 mg/DL

MAJOR RISK FACTORS THAT INFLUENCE LDL CHOLESTEROL GOALS

- Smoking
- Hypertension (BP $\geq$ 140/90 or taking antihypertensive medication
- Low HDL cholesterol (men <40 mg/dl, women <50 mg/dl)
- Family history of premature CHD (CHD in first degree <65 yr. and female, < 55yr.
- Age (men $\geq$ 45 yr., women $\geq$ 55 yr.)

SOLUBLE FIBER and LOWERING LDL CHOLESTEROL

A diet high in soluble fiber has been shown to reduce LDL cholesterol. Soluble fiber is found in plant foods and because it is not absorbed in the intestine, it binds cholesterol in the intestine and removes it from the body. You may be able to reduce your LDL cholesterol by eating 5 to 10 grams of soluble fiber by choosing foods that have at least 2-3 grams each.

Water-soluble fiber foods include:

- Avocado
- Chia seeds, flax seeds, chia seeds, nuts
- Chickpeas, black, kidney, pinto, navy, soy and lima beans
- Cooked barley, oatmeal, oat bran, quinoa, psyllium
- Brussel sprouts, cabbage, carrots, green beans, okra, onions, beans, parsnips, turnips
- Sweet potatoes, potatoes
- Bananas, guava, oranges, peaches, pears, apricots, plums, figs, dried apricots, prunes, blackberries, and raspberries

LOWERING YOUR CHOLESTEROL:

- Work with a dietitian to develop an individualized meal plan
- Use less oil, butter, margarine, and other fats
- Choose low-fat dairy instead of full fats
- Eat smaller servings of meat, fish, and poultry
- Eat more fruits and vegetables, 5 servings or more per day
- Maintain a healthy weight or lose weight; just 5%-7% weight loss helps
- Choose whole grains such as oatmeal, whole-wheat bread, brown rice, quinoa, and barley
- Exercise for 30 minutes most days
- Know your medications and their interactions
- Quit smoking
- Use food products that contain plant sterols
- Include unsalted tree nuts (almonds, walnuts, pistachios), peanuts, and seeds
- 8-12 oz. per week of seafood high in Omega-3, such as salmon, mackerel, sardines and tuna

TYPES OF FAT

Trans-fatty acids are formed by adding hydrogen atoms to an unsaturated fat creating an unnatural trans-fat. Common sources of trans-fatty acids are partially hydrogenated vegetable oils found in stick margarines and deep-fried fast foods. These facts are often used to prolong the shelf-life of packaged foods such as crackers, potato chips, and cookies. Trans-fats can raise LDL levels and lower HDL levels. Studies have shown that trans-fats can increase the risk for cardiovascular disease.

Since 2006, trans fats have been required to be listed on food labels in the U.S. Many companies have worked to remove trans fats from their products. Since the FDA allows products with <0.5 grams trans fats to claim 0 grams trans fats, the labeling may be misleading. Check the nutrition label and look for 0 grams of trans fat. Then read the ingredient list. If the words hydrogenation or partial hydrogenation appear, count that food as having at least 0.5 grams trans fats.

TRANS-FATS AND HYDROGENATION

There is no recommended safe level for trans-fatty acids. Though some trans fats occur naturally in foods, most are the result of adding hydrogen to liquid oil. This chemical change hardens the oil, a process called hydrogenation.

Hydrogenation causes these oils to become like saturated fats and lengthens the shelf life of food products and can improve taste and texture. However, research shows that eating foods with hydrogenated oils increases the risk of heart disease.

Effect on Cholesterol: Trans fats and hydrogenated fats can increase LDL cholesterol and triglycerides and decrease HDL cholesterol, the "good" cholesterol.

Food Sources of Trans Fats

- Vegetable shortening
- Some margarines
- Commercially prepared foods and fried foods like potato chips, crackers, cookies, and cakes

SATURATED FATS

Generally, saturated fats are solid at room temperature. You can find the grams of saturated fat on packaged food labels. The U.S.

Dietary Guidelines 2020-2025 is recommending the restriction of saturated fat intake to be <10% of calories to reduce cardiovascular disease.

Dietary saturated fat remains controversial. Some studies have found that saturated fats do not contribute to cardiovascular disease but have found their intake to be protective against stroke. It has also been found that whole-fat dairy, dark chocolate, and unprocessed meats, all high in saturated fats are associated with increase in cardiovascular benefits.

Food Sources of Saturated fat:

- Meat
- Cheese Processed foods
- Eggs
- Dairy Products
- Palm Oil and Coconut oil
- Butter
- Lard
- Most Processed foods

Foods High in Saturated Fat and Cholesterol

- Meats
  - Some cuts of beef, pork, lamb
  - Regular ground beef (choose 90% lean)
  - Spareribs
  - Organ meats – liver, kidneys
  - Fried chicken, fried fish, and fried shellfish
  - Bologna, salami, sausage, and hot dogs
  - All visible fat on meat is saturated, trim it off when possible
  - Poultry skin. Remove skin after cooking.
  - Not all red meats are high in fat. Many red meats are lean and can be worked into your diet. Check out the list of lean meat choices at the end of this chapter.

- Eggs
  - 1 egg has about 213 mg cholesterol, all of it in the yolk. But the cholesterol found in egg yolks may not be as harmful as once thought. But for those with high cholesterol, limiting egg yolks to about 2 per week is still recommended.

- Dairy Products
  - Milk (both whole and 2%). Choose low fat varieties
  - Whole milk yogurt and yogurt beverages. Choose low fat varieties
  - Regular cheese -- look for part- skim or skim, for example mozzarella and ricotta
  - Cream, half and half, whipping cream, and nondairy creamer
  - Whipped topping
  - Sour cream. Choose low-fat, fat-free, or just skip it if only a condiment

Foods High in Saturated Fat and Cholesterol

- Fats and Oils
  - Coconut oil
  - Palm kernel oil
  - Butter and margarine
  - Lard
  - Bacon fat
  - Salad dressings
- Fried Foods
  - Anything deep-fried such as fried chicken, French fries, tortilla chips
- Creamed Foods
  - Creamy sauces, gravies, and soups
  - Substitute lower fat ingredients when preparing these foods at home.
- Commercially Prepared Baked Foods and Desserts
  - Many of these foods are made with fats such as p a l m oil or coconut oil. These oils are less expensive for manufacturers to use. Make your own dessert or enjoy fruit at the end of the meal.

Saturated Fat in Lean Meat Choices

Lean Red Meat Cuts*	Calories	Sat. Fat (grams)	Total Fat (grams)
Eye Round Roast and Steak*	144	1.4	4.0
Sirloin Tip Side Steak	143	1.6	4.1
Top Round Roast and Steak*	157	1.6	4.6
Bottom Round Roast and Steak*	139	1.7	4.9
Top Sirloin Steak	156	1.9	4.9
Brisket, Flat Half	167	1.9	5.1
95% Lean Ground Beef	139	2.3	5.1
Round Tip Roast and Steak*	148	1.9	5.3
Round Steak	154	1.9	5.3
Shank Cross Cuts	171	1.9	5.4
Chunk Shoulder Pot Roast	147	1.8	5.7

Lean Red Meat Cuts*	Calories	Sat. Fat (grams)	Total Fat (grams)
Sirloin Tip Center Roast and Steak*	150	2.1	5.8
Chuck Shoulder Steak	161	1.9	6.0
Bottom Round (Western Griller) Steak	155	2.2	6.0
Top Loin (Strip) Steak	161	2.6	6.0
Shoulder Petite Tender and Medallions*	150	2.4	6.1
Flank Steak	158	2.6	6.3
Shoulder Center (Ranch) Steak	155	2.4	6.5
Tri-Tip Roast and Steak*	158	2.6	7.1
Tenderloin Roast and Steak	170	2.7	7.1
T-Bone Steak	172	3.0	8.2
Lean White Meat Cuts*			
Pork Tenderloin, separated lean white meat only	104	1.0	2.8
Skinless Chicken Thigh	188	2.7	9.8
Skinless Chicken Breast	148	0.9	3.2
White Tuna Canned in Water	109	0.7	2.5
Salmon	175	2.1	10.5

Approx. cooked protein portions are 4 ounces.

** Cuts combined for illustration purposes.

Source: U.S. Department of Agriculture, Agricultural Research Service, 2008. USDA Nutrient Database for Standard Reference, Release 21.

[1] Source: U.S. Department of Agriculture, Agricultural Research Service, 2009. USDA Nutrient Database for Standard Reference, Release 22.

MONOUNSATURATED FATS

Monounsaturated fats are liquid at room temperature but become solid when refrigerated. Use these types of fats when preparing your foods.

Effect on Cholesterol: Monounsaturated fats seem to reduce LDL cholesterol and total cholesterol and keep HDL the same.

Food Sources of Monounsaturated fat:

- Canola Oil
- Peanut Oil
- Olive Oil
- Sunflower Oil
- Almond Oil
- Sesame Oil
- Almonds*
- Peanut Butter
- Avocados

Almonds* are also an excellent source of the antioxidant alpha-tocopherol from Vitamin E. This antioxidant has been shown to prevent cholesterol from sticking to artery walls. One ounce of almonds (about 23 almonds) has 160 calories and 7.4 mg of alpha-tocopherol. That is about half the calories of 2 ounces of potato chips or a candy bar, making almonds and other nuts a good snack choice.

POLYUNSATURATED FATS

Defined: Polyunsaturated fats are also liquid at room temperature, but unlike monounsaturated fats, these remain liquid even when refrigerated. Polyunsaturated fats are probably the most commonly used fats in the family kitchen.

Monounsaturated fats are liquid at room temperature but become solid when refrigerated. Use these types of fats when preparing your foods.

Effect on Cholesterol: Monounsaturated fats seem to reduce LDL cholesterol and total cholesterol and keep HDL the same.

- Canola Oil
- Peanut Oil
- Olive Oil
- Sunflower Oil
- Almond Oil
- Sesame Oil
- Almonds*
- Peanut Butter
- Avocados

Effect on Cholesterol: Polyunsaturated fats are known to lower LDL cholesterol, which is good, but they can also lower HDL cholesterol, which is not so good.

Food Sources of Polyunsaturated fat:

- Corn Oil,
- Soybean Oil,
- Safflower Oil,
- Sunflower Oil.

Walnuts- have also been shown in studies to reduce cholesterol and LDL levels, Margarine- yet if eaten in large quantities may also have a negative effect by reducing HDL.

OMEGA-3 FATTY ACIDS

These are a type of polyunsaturated fat that also provide protection against heart disease. There are three types of omega-3 fatty acids: alpha-linolenic acid (ALA), eicosatetraenoic acid (EPA), and docosa-hexaenoic acid (DHA). The body uses EPA and DHA more efficiently, whereas ALA requires further conversion. DHA and EPA are found in algae, which fish and seafood eat.

Effect on Cholesterol: Omega-3 fatty acids can lower the risk of heart disease by making the blood less "sticky" and less likely to clot. They can also lower triglycerides. For heart protection, the recommendation for omega-3 fatty acids per day is 1 gram. However, for lowering triglycerides, 2 to 4 grams per day have been shown to be beneficial.

Food Sources of Omega-3 Fatty Acids:

- Chia Seeds
- Pumpkin Seeds
- Walnuts
- Flaxseed
- Canola Oil
- Soy
- Spinach
- Brussel Sprouts
- Kale
- Cauliflower
- Broccoli
- Fatty fish such as salmon, oysters, mackerel, albacore tuna, and sardines - at least 2 servings of fatty fish per week are recommended

PHYTOSTEROLS

Phytosterols are also known as plant sterols. These cholesterol-like substances naturally occur in plants such as grains, nuts and legumes, vegetable oils, vegetables, and fruits. Though similar in structure to animal cholesterol, phytosterols help lower blood cholesterol levels. At the end of this chapter there are two charts, which can help you identify which products contain plant sterols.

Effect on Cholesterol: They slow or prevent the absorption of cholesterol from food and the cholesterol produced by the liver, preventing cholesterol from entering your blood. Although many foods on the market contain phytosterols, long-term studies are not available yet to know their long-term effects.

Food Sources of Phytosterols:

- Promise Activ Spread
- Take Control
- Benecol
- Smart Balance
- Health Valley Heart Wise Cereal and Granola Bars
- Minute Maid Premium Heart Wise Orange Juice
- Kroger Active Lifestyle Fat Free Milk

The dietary supplement CholestOff by Nature Made blends plant sterols and stanols inhibiting the absorption of cholesterol from food causing some of it to pass through the body.

Oils (1 tbsp.)	Total Plant Sterols
Corn Oil	100.0 - 133.3
Cottonseed Oil	24.0 - 29.2
Olive Oil (Extra Virgin)	10.7 - 11.1
Palm Oil	3.6 - 4.5
Rapeseed Oil	35.0 - 102.0
Canola Oil	89.1 - 91.3
Rice Bran Oil	77.6
Soybean Oil	30.1 - 44.7
Sunflower Oil	27.5 - 53.3
Cereal Grains (.25 cup)	
Rye	38.4 - 46.5
Wheat	28.9 - 33.1
Oats	12.8 - 20.3
Barley	29.3 - 41.5
Vegetables (1 cup)	
Corn	274.1
Brussel Sprouts	37.8
Broccoli	35.5
Cauliflower	40.0
Carrot	20.5
Potato	14.0
Apple	16.3
Orange	43.2
Legumes (.75 cup)	
Chickpea	174.8 - 188.9
Lentil	160.8 - 177.0
While Bean	155.0 - 172.6
Peanut	52.3 - 55.4

Nuts and Seeds	
Almond	25.2 - 26.8
Hazelnut	23.0 - 24.5
Pistachio	48.2 - 50.5
Sunflower Seed	39.3 - 41.7
Walnut	16.0 - 16.8

Published with permission from the Diabetes Care and Education Dietetic Practice Group of the Academy of Nutrition and Dietetics: Rideout TC, Lun B. Plant Sterols in the Management of Dyslipidemia in Patients with Diabetes. *On the Cutting Edge.* 2010;31(6):13-17.

Spreads	Total Plant Sterols
Benecol - Regular & Light Spreads	850 mg/tbsp.
Take Control - Promise Active Spreads (Buttery & Light)	1,000 mg/tbsp.
Beverages	
Minute Maid - Heart Wise Orange Juice	1,000 mg/8 fl. oz
Milks	
Rice Dream - Heartwise (Original & Vanilla)	650 mg/8 fl. oz
Silk - Heart Health Soy Milk	650 mg/8 fl. oz
Giant Eagle - Fat Free Milk	400 mg/8 fl. oz
Kroger - Active Lifestyle Fat-Free Milk	400 mg/8 fl. oz
Cheese	
Lifeline - Lifetime Low Fat Cheese	650 mg/8 fl. oz
Chews	
Quest - Cardio Chews (Chewy, Chocolate)	400 mg/chew
Benecol - Smart Chews	850 mg/chew

Baked Goods

Kroger - Active Lifestyle Bread	800 mg/serving
Krusteaz - Healthy Start Pancakes and Waffles	650 mg/serving
Vitamuffin - Dark Chocolate Pomegranate Vitatops	400 mg/top

Pastas

Racconto - Heart Health Pastas	400 mg/serving

Published with permission from the Diabetes Care and Education Dietetic Practice Group of the Academy of Nutrition and Dietetics: Rideout TC, Lun B. Plant Sterols in the Management of Dyslipidemia in Patients with Diabetes. *On the Cutting Edge.* 2010;31(6):13-17.7.

KNOW YOUR OILS

In 2018, the FDA approved one cardiovascular health claim for oils and heart health – extra-virgin olive oil, certain types of algal, canola, sunflower and safflower oils. To meet the criteria, the oil must be at least 70% oleic acid. FDA states: "Supportive but not conclusive scientific evidence suggests that daily consumption of about 1 ½ tablespoons (20 grams) of oils containing high levels of oleic acid may reduce the risk of coronary heart disease." FDA also said that these oils "should replace fats and oils higher in saturated fat and not increase the total number of calories you eat daily".

In addition to nutrition, choose oils for flavor and consider their cooking characteristics. The smoke point refers to the temperature at which cooking oil breaks down and will begin to smoke or flame, and both flavor and nutrition are compromised. Another concern is that high cooking temperatures of unsaturated oils can convert them to saturated oils. For this reason, deep-frying is not recommended.

THE LOW DOWN ON OILS

Extra-Virgin Olive Oil	Contains mostly monounsaturated fat. It has a light, peppery flavor and a low smoke point. The low smoke point makes this oil better for a quick sauté of fish or other meats, and even better as a dressing for topping off salads and vegetables.
Olive Oil	Good for sautéing or adding to salads, vegetables.
Canola Oil	Contains mostly monounsaturated fat with the least amount of saturated fat of the oils. It has a neutral flavor and a moderate smoke point making it good for sautéing and baking.
Peanut Oil	Contains about 50% monounsaturated fat and about 30% polyunsaturated fat. This oil is good for sautéing and frying. Has a high smoke point.
Corn Oil & Vegetable Oil	High in polyunsaturated fat it has a high smoke point, which makes this oil good for frying.
Sunflower & Safflower Oil	High in polyunsaturated fat and it is good for deep frying and high heat cooking.
Flaxseed Oil	Best used for salad dressings. Has a low smoke point.
Grapeseed Oil	Has a moderately high smoke point. Good for sauté and frying. Good for salad dressings and dips.

Omega-3's & MERCURY

Fish is a great source of protein and is low in calories and saturated fat. It is also high in the omega-3 fats EPA and DHA. Wild fish tends to have more Omega-3s while fish like swordfish and mackerel may accumulate heavy metals. The 2020-2025 Dietary Guidelines recommend 8 to 12 ounces of seafood per week for Americans. And in 2019, the FDA and the Environmental Protection Agency (EPA) revised its advice for women who may become pregnant, pregnant women, nursing mothers, and young children, saying eating 8 to 12 ounces of fish low in mercury is beneficial. According to the FDA and EPA, most fish in grocery stores are lower in mercury and safe for pregnant women and children at 8 to 12 ounces per week. These include shrimp, pollock, salmon, canned light tuna, tilapia, catfish and cod. Types of fish to avoid because of potential mercury content include tilefish from the Gulf of Mexico, shark, swordfish and king mackerel.

Following is a list of fish and their mercury content.

Avoid	Omega-3 Fatty Acids (grams per 3 oz)	Mean mercury level in parts per million (ppm)
Swordfish	0.97	0.97
Shark	0.83	0.99
King Mackerel	0.36	0.73
Tilefish (golden bass or golden snapper)	0.90	1.45

Top 10 Healthy Fish Based on Omega-3 & Mercury Levels		
	Omega-3 Fatty Acids (grams per 3 oz)	Mean mercury level In parts per million (ppm)
Canned Tune (light)	0.17 - 0.24	0.12
Shrimp	0.29	Below detection levels
Pollock	0.45	0.06
Salmon (fresh, frozen)	1.1 - 1.9	0.01
Cod	0.15 - 0.24	0.11
Catfish	0.22 - 0.30	0.05
Clams	0.25	Below detection levels
Flounder or Sole	0.48	0.05
Crabs	0.27 - 0.40	0.06
Scallops	0.18 - 0.34	0.05

Source for above tables: Natural Resource Defense Council, adapted from FDA guidelines.

Albacore ("white") tuna has more mercury than canned light tuna. So, when choosing your two meals of fish and shellfish, you may eat up to 6 ounces (one average meal) of albacore tuna per week.

NUTTY NUTRITION

Tree nuts are rich in protein, minerals, fiber, phytonutrients, anti-oxidants, vitamin E, manganese, thiamin, phosphorus, and magnesium. The FDA approved a Qualified Health claim stating: Eating 1.5 ounces per day of most nuts or 2 tbs. nut butters several times each week as a part of a diet low in saturated fat and cholesterol may reduce the risk of heart disease.

Nuts	Number of Nuts	Calories	Protein (grams)	Fat (grams)	Saturated Fat (grams)
Almonds	23	190	6	14	1
Brazil Nuts	6	190	4	19	4
Cashews	18	160	4	13	3
Hazel Nuts	21	180	4	17	1.5
Macadamia	11	200	2	22	3.5
Pecans	19	200	3	20	2
Pine Nuts	167	190	4	20	1.5
Pistachios	49	190	6	13	1.5
Walnuts	14	185	4	18	2

BUTTER OR MARGARINE?

Butter, if used in moderation, should present no problem. Butter has more saturated fat, and cholesterol. Whipped butter has fewer calories, fat, saturated fat, and cholesterol because air is whipped into the product during processing. Light butter has even lower calories, fat, saturated fat, and cholesterol because some of the fat is replaced by water or gelatin.

The best choice would be whipped margarines that contain plant stanols, which are natural substances that lower cholesterol levels by decreasing its absorption. These would include: Smart Balance, Benecol, and Unilever's Take Control margarines.

Spread	Calories	Fat (g)	Sat. Fat (g)	Cholesterol
Stick Butter	100	11	7	30
Whipped Butter	70	8	5	20
Light Butter	60	7	2	7
Butter/Oil Blend	100	11	4	15

Spread	Calories	Fat (g)	Sat. Fat (g)	Cholesterol
Light Butter/Oil Blend	50	5	2	5
Stick Margarine	100	11	2	0
Whipped Margarine	70	7	1-2	0
Light Whipped Margarine	50	5.5	1.5	0
Trans Free Stick for Baking Margarine	80	9	2.5	0
Plant Sterol Margarine	80	9	2.5	0
Plant Sterol Margarine Light	50	5	1.5	0

Answers to Cholesterol Questions:

1. True
2. True
3. False. HDL is the "good" cholesterol that protects against heart disease. High levels are desirable.
4. False. You should lower the total amount of fat in your diet and lower the amount of saturated fat consumed
5. False. Dietary cholesterol is found in animal foods. Fruits and vegetables contain no cholesterol.
6. False. Cholesterol is formed in the liver.
7. True

SODIUM: IT'S NATURALLY SALTY

Sodium Questions: Test your knowledge by answering True or False to the questions below concerning sodium in your diet.

1. The amount of sodium I eat is only a concern if I have high blood pressure or a family history of high blood pressure.
2. We should try to consume less than 2,300 mg of sodium a day.
3. A teaspoon of salt contains about 3,000 mg of sodium.
4. Most sodium in our diet comes from processed foods.
5. A high sodium intake increases the risk for high blood pressure and heart disease.

It's hard to imagine a meal without salt. Salt enhances the flavor of food, and without it, many foods taste bland. But this treasured spice has been feeling the pinch as it has been linked to high blood pressure and heavily processed foods and fast foods. Many Americans have acquired a taste for foods high in sodium and are eating more than necessary.

Eating fresh, minimally processed foods is the easiest way to limit sodium. Eating healthy includes looking at the amount of salt in your diet.

It may seem impossible to avoid sodium. Most foods naturally contain it. Prepared foods contain added sodium, and then there's the sodium we add while cooking and eating. Here's the breakdown on sodium in our diet:

- 5% added during cooking
- 6% added during eating
- 12% found naturally in foods
- 77% found in prepared and processed food

WHY DO WE NEED SODIUM?

- Sodium maintains the balance of fluids in the body.
- Sodium transmits nerve impulses.
- Sodium helps with contraction and relaxation of muscles

HOW MUCH IS ENOUGH?

The average American consumes as much as 5,000 mg a day, and yet The National Academy of Sciences' National Academy of Medicine states that 1,500 mg of sodium per day is adequate for good health. The new 2020-2025 Dietary Guidelines recommend limiting salt intake to 2,300 mg a day: about 1 teaspoon of salt. Recent studies show that sodium doesn't increase health risks unless intake is greater than five grams daily.

Some experts link high sodium intake to hypertension, cardiovascular disease, kidney disease, and stroke. Yet there are some who disagree. Studies show that only in communities with over five grams of sodium daily was there a direct link between intake and heart attack and stroke. Researchers also found that when potassium was higher, there was a decrease in major cardiovascular events. Foods high in potassium include bananas, oranges, cantaloupe, kiwi, avocados, spinach, Brussel sprouts, sweet and white potatoes, nuts, and beans.

The DASH and Mediterranean diets are lower in sodium and have been shown to reduce blood pressure. The Dietary Approaches to Stop Hypertension Study (DASH) found that blood pressure was lowered in participants who cut their sodium intake to 1,500 mg per day. The DASH diet recommends eating fresh unprocessed foods and foods high in potassium, magnesium, and calcium which can counterbalance the effects of sodium.

So, the sodium debate continues, but we know it does matter, especially for people with high blood pressure, chronic kidney disease and other health issues. We recommend you eat more fresh and unprocessed food and explore herbs and spices that boost flavor—and use salt in moderation.

BECOME A SODIUM SLEUTH

The biggest contributor to sodium in the diet is restaurant and processed foods. If you eat out frequently, you're probably getting too much sodium.

When eating out, especially at fast food and fast casual restaurants, check the nutrition information for dishes on restaurant websites.

For packaged foods, start with the Nutrition Facts Label on canned and packaged foods. Packages and processed foods often contain large amounts of sodium, especially soups. Look for labels that say, "reduced sodium".

The Percent Daily Value allows you to compare products and lists the amount of sodium. A DV of 5% or less is low; 20% DV or more is high. Labels provide the sodium content in milligrams for a single serving based on a 2,000-calorie diet. The Daily Values would differ for individuals whose calorie intake is less or more than a 2,000-calorie diet.

LABEL LINGO

The number of lower sodium products has more than doubled in the past 5 years. Look for these strictly defined terms on the front of food packaging.

Salt Free (or Sodium Free)	Less than 5 mg sodium per serving
No Salt Added	No salt added during processing; but does not mean sodium free
Very Low Sodium	35 mg or less sodium per serving
Low Sodium	140 mg or less per serving
Light in Sodium	50% less sodium than the regular product, restricted to those foods that have more than 40 calories per serving or more than 3 grams of fat per serving
Less Sodium or Reduced Sodium	At least 25% less sodium than the regular product. These foods may still have a significant amount of sodium.

BEYOND FOOD

Some over-the-counter drugs contain sodium. Be sure to read the label before taking drugs such as antacids. If an antacid contains 5 mg or more of sodium per serving, it must be listed on the label. Watch out for the word "soda," referring to sodium bicarbonate or baking soda. These products are made of sodium compounds.

REDUCING YOUR SODIUM

Your goal is to stay within the recommended 2,300 mg of sodium daily. Balancing a high sodium meal with a meal that is fresh and unprocessed will help you stay within that limit. Lowering salt intake doesn't mean you have to forfeit flavor. Start with small changes, they really do add up.

When adding salt, either during cooking or at the table, these quantities give you an idea of the sodium content for each serving:

¼ teaspoon salt	575 mg sodium
½ teaspoon salt	1,150 mg sodium
¾ teaspoon salt	1,725 mg sodium
1 teaspoon salt	2,300 mg sodium
1 teaspoon baking soda	1,000 mg sodium

TIPS FOR REDUCING SODIUM:

1. Buy fresh or frozen vegetables. If you buy canned vegetables, look for items without added salt or drain and rinse the vegetables before cooking.

2. Limit canned, cured, processed, or smoked meats and packaged and convenience foods.

3. Limit foods that are packed in brine: pickles, olives, sauerkraut, and pickled vegetables.

4. Limit condiments that are high in sodium: soy sauce, garlic salt, bouillon cubes, bottled marinades, soup bases, and Worcestershire sauce. Instead, use spices and herbs to enhance flavor.

5. Limit salty snacks like chips, pretzels, salted nuts and crackers. Look for low-sodium products and choose unsalted nuts and seeds.

6. Cut back on fast foods. Check the nutrition content of fast foods online. Often, one item will exceed the daily requirement for sodium.

7. Cook without salt, then taste and add it after cooking if needed. Cook rice, pasta, and hot cereals without salt.

8. Read labels for sodium content. Keep an eye on the number of servings you would consume to determine if the product is safe for you to consume.

Noteworthy: Sea salt and kosher salt contain the same amount of sodium by weight as table salt, but often are more flavorful. So still use in moderation.

Spices, flavorings, vegetables, and herbs can be used to naturally enhance the flavors of food. Sea salt and kosher salt still contain the same amount of sodium by weight, but often are more flavorful. Experiment by utilizing the following guide and find the combinations you prefer. Two websites that you can check for more information are: www.spiceadvice.com and nhlbi.nih.gov/hbp/prevent/sodium/flavor.htm

MANAGING THE MENU

1. Limit foods with sauces.

2. Avoid breaded and fried foods, which can be high in sodium. Choose baked or broiled meats and fish.

3. Choose salad over soup. Soups are usually high in sodium.

4. Ask if the dishes can be prepared without added salt.

5. Choose oil and vinegar or lemon juice for salads. Or ask for dressings on the side.

6. Cutback on the condiments. Choose fresh tomato, lettuce, and cucumber for sandwiches rather than olives and pickles. Go easy on condiments; ketchup, sauces, cheese, and mayonnaise are hidden sources of sodium.

REPLACE SALT WITH HERBS AND SPICES

Beef	Allspice, bay leaf, caraway seeds, curry powder, dill, dry mustard, ginger, mushrooms, onions, onion flakes, pepper, sage, thyme, and tomatoes
Fish	Allspice, curry powder, Dijon mustard, dill, ginger, green pepper, honey, mushrooms, mustard, lemon, lemon pepper, tarragon, thyme, and tomatoes
Lamb	Curry powder, dill, mint, and sage
Pork	Basil, caraway, Dijon mustard, dry mustard, honey mustard, nutmeg, rosemary, and tarragon
Poultry	Bay leaf, dill, curry powder, ginger, green pepper, lemon, lemon pepper, marjoram, mushrooms, poultry seasoning, rosemary, sage, tarragon, thyme, and tomatoes
Veal	Bay leaf, tomatoes
Carrots	Ginger, marjoram, oregano, paprika, rosemary, sage, tarragon, and thyme
Corn	Cumin, curry powder, onion, paprika, and parsley
Green Beans	Dill, curry powder, lemon juice, marjoram, oregano, tarragon, and thyme
Greens	Onion, garlic, and pepper
Peas	Ginger, marjoram, onion, parsley, and sage
Potatoes	Dill, garlic, onion, paprika, parsley, and sage
Summer Squash	Cloves, curry powder, marjoram, nutmeg, rosemary, and sage
Winter Squash	Cinnamon, ginger, nutmeg, and onion
Tomatoes	Basil, bay leaf, dill, marjoram, onion, oregano, parsley, and pepper

TYPES OF SALT	
Table Salts	• Salt (plain & iodized)
Reduced Sodium Products	• Salt substitute is 100% potassium chloride • Morton Lite Salt Mixture is 50% sodium chloride (NaCl) and 50% potassium chloride (KCl) • Morton Salt Balance Salt Blend is 75% NaCl and 25% KCl • Salt Sense is 100% sodium. The salt crystal is puffed, making it bigger than a normal crystal. There is 33% less salt in the container.
Gourmet and Specialty Salts	• Kosher Salt • Sea Salt (Fine & Coarse) • Popcorn Salt • Canning & Pickling Salt • Ice Cream Salt • Himalayan Pink Sea salt, smoked salt, black salt and grey salt. Contain the same amount of sodium as table salt, but they have a more complex flavor.
Seasoned and Flavored Salts	• Morton's Nature's Seasons Seasoning Blend • Garlic Salt • Seasoned Salt • Hot Salt • Sausage & Meat Loaf Seasoning Mix

Potassium is the mineral substituted for sodium in salt substitutes. It has an unpleasant metallic aftertaste. If you have kidney disease and limit your potassium intake you should avoid this salt substitute. By cooking with extra spices, you can mask some of this flavor. Morton Salt Balance Salt Blend is only 25% potassium chloride (KCl). You get a 25% reduction in sodium and can't taste the KCl.

Remember that sodium is an essential nutrient. However, moderate salt intake is part of a healthy diet and lifestyle. So… Are you salting before tasting?

Answers to Sodium Questions:

1. False. As sodium intake increases so does blood pressure.
2. False. The daily sodium recommendation is less than 2,300 mg per day.
3. False. One teaspoon of salt contains 2,300 mg of sodium.
4. True
5. True

FIBER FARE

"The only way to keep your health is to eat what you don't want, drink what you don't want, and do what you druther not."

— *Mark Twain*

Fiber **Questions:** Test your knowledge of dietary fiber.

1. The average American eats only 10-15 grams of fiber daily.
2. Fiber should be added gradually to the diet along with plenty of fluids.
3. Some people may experience side effects when increasing their fiber intake.
4. Eating high fiber foods will cause weight gain.
5. Women should eat 15 grams of fiber daily and men 20 grams.

We often turn our noses up at the mention of high fiber foods. Yet many high fiber foods taste good, fit easily into a daily meal plan, and make us feel fuller between meals. High fiber foods are an important part of a healthy diet that shouldn't be ignored.

Fiber is too often the overlooked sibling in the nutrient family, despite research showing its many health benefits. Americans just aren't eating enough whole grains and other high fiber foods. The average American consumes less than 15 grams of fiber a day.

The National Academy of Sciences recommends 25 grams of fiber daily for women up to age 50 (slightly lower for women after age 50) and 38 grams a day for men.

FIBER FACTS

Dietary fiber is the carbohydrate portion of plant foods that our bodies cannot digest. There are two kinds of dietary fiber: soluble and insoluble. Most foods contain some of both. Soluble fiber dissolves in water to form a gel-like, viscous substance. It can be found in oats, peas, beans, apples, citrus, carrots, and barley. Insoluble fiber increases the movement of material through the digestive system. It is found in whole wheat products, wheat bran, most vegetables, and nuts. Another type of insoluble fiber is resistant starch, which "resists" digestion. Good sources include bananas, lentils, beans, and whole grains. Hi-maize® resistant starch is made from special corn. It is added to certain products like Racconto pastas to increase fiber. It can also be purchased and added to cereals, smoothies, and baked products. For more information about resistant starches, visit www.healthline.com/nutrition/resistant-starch-101.

WHY IS FIBER GOOD FOR ME?

Fiber can help lower cholesterol, especially when combined with a low-fat diet. Researchers at Harvard University found that men who ate about 29 grams of fiber a day had a 40% reduction in heart attacks compared with men with a low fiber intake.

Fiber alters large bowel function by increasing stool bulk and decreasing the amount of time it takes to move through the bowel. This reduces the exposure of the bowel to carcinogens and protects against cancers of the colon and rectum. Fiber promotes regularity and may reduce the risk of diverticulitis—inflammation of small pouches in the lining of the colon.

Recommended adequate intake of Fiber: 38 grams for men and 25 grams for women per day.

Foods high in fiber will give you a sense of satiety —"full feeling" between meals — and aid in weight loss. A study published in the February 2011 *Journal of Nutrition* involved two groups of mice that had their calories restricted and then could eat as much as they wanted. One group of mice had fiber added to their diet. That group lost almost 4% of body fat. The other group regained their weight. So, adding more fiber to your diet may reduce the consumption of high-calorie foods, making it easier to lose weight.

WHOLE GRAINS

A good place to start to increase fiber intake is whole grains. They are delicious, versatile, and fit any level of cooking skill. Whole grains are high in fiber and vitamins, especially B vitamins, are low in fat, and are cholesterol free. To get the benefits of all these nutrients, all three parts of the grain must be consumed. White flour, white rice, and other refined grains have had the bran and germ removed, leaving only the middle, starchy layer, which is devoid of most nutrients. Processing removes approximately 25% of the grain's protein and as many as 17 nutrients. Some are added back, "enriching" the grains, but not all and not to the same levels. To get the total benefit, cut back on the refined grains and consume more whole grains. Try making at least half your grains whole grains. For cooking ideas, see *Whole Grains for Busy People* by Lorna Sass.

WHOLE GRAIN KERNELS

Parts of the grain

1. Outer bran: Rich in fiber
2. Middle, starchy endosperm: Makes up about 80% of the grain
3. Inner germ: Packed with nutrients

Types of Whole Grains:

Whole Wheat, Oats, Barley (not pearled), Corn (not degerminated), Buckwheat, Bulgur, Quinoa, Farro, Freekeh, Amaranth, Brown and Wild Rice, Millet, Rye, Sorghum, Spelt, Teff, Triticale, Kamut®, and Einkorn. Whole grains contain not only fiber but also hundreds of phytochemicals (such as phytoestrogens), antioxidants, phenols, vitamins, and minerals (such as Vitamin E and selenium). These all play a role in disease prevention. Many compounds in grains, including antioxidants, have been shown to lower the risk for cardiovascular disease and some forms of cancer.

READING FOOD LABELS

Don't be fooled by color. Just because a product has a caramel or brown color does not mean it is whole grain. For example, rye and pumpernickel bread seldom provide much fiber and are not whole grain products, despite their dark color. The words "natural" and "organic" do not mean a food is made from whole grains. Look for the words "whole wheat flour" on the ingredient list to be certain the product was made from the whole grain.

Also, the number of grams of fiber on the label does not mean the food is whole grain. Whole grain products do have 2 grams of fiber or more in one serving; however, to determine if a product is truly whole grain, look for the words "whole wheat" or "whole grain." Generally, a good source of fiber contains 2.5 or more grams of fiber per serving. Check the label and ingredient list for fiber information.

Some foods contain inulin (aka chicory root extract), modified wheat starch, polydextrose, and maltodextrin. Inulin is added as "food" to prebiotics, to help boost intestinal flora. Modified wheat starch is used in white, high fiber pasta, but there are no studies to date regarding the health benefit of this product. Although these are soluble fibers, they are not viscous or "gummy" and don't lower cholesterol. These types of fiber are referred to in the world of food science as "isolated fiber" and are found in ice cream, yogurt, fat-free half and half, white pastas, and some breakfast bars.

Naturally grown foods typically contain whole grains and most processed foods do not. However, there are some products that have added processed fiber, like tapioca fiber, and they are a great healthy alternative. The fiber in these processed foods will still act as a laxative in preventing constipation, but the antioxidants and phytonutrients that are present in whole grains will be missing.

Some foods also contain functional fibers: cellulose, chitin, oligo-fructose, fructooligosaccharides, lignin, pectins, psyllium, and inulin (aka chicory root). They are found in fruits and vegetables and added to foods to increase fiber content. Inulin is often added to foods such as candy bars, snack foods, and chocolate milk. But know that too much Inulin could cause gas and bloating.

FINDING THE FIBER

Adults should try to eat 25 – 35 grams of fiber each day. With a little planning and smart shopping, you can easily hit that target in meals and snacks.

BREAKFAST

- Look for high-fiber cereals such as General Mill's Fiber One or Kellogg's All-Bran. They can contain as much as 13 grams of fiber in one serving.
- Add fruit, chia seeds or flax seeds to oatmeal or high-fiber cereal and you could have half of your daily requirement in one meal.
- Try a 100% Whole Grain English muffin or bread and add avocado. A third of a medium avocado (50 g) has 3 grams of fiber and 80 calories.
- Try a homemade bran muffin with a piece of fruit.

LUNCH

- Look for Brownberry's Whole Grain Bread with Double Fiber/ Extra Fiber, which has 6 grams of fiber per slice. That's an easy 12 grams for a sandwich. Bump up the fiber even more by adding greens such as lettuce, spinach or arugula and tomatoes to it.
- Add fresh fruit for lunch and you'll have 14 grams for the meal.
- Skip the chips and eat a small salad or raw vegetables with your sandwich or as a snack.

SNACK

- Bring raw chopped vegetables and low-fat dip.
- Grab a piece of fruit instead of heading to the vending machine.
- Bring a small container (1/4-1/2 cup) of nuts from home.
- A 100-calorie bag of popcorn

DINNER

- Beans: Excellent source of fiber. They have soluble fiber which can help lower cholesterol.
  Kidney beans, chickpeas, black beans, pinto beans, lentils, and black-eyed peas can be added to a salad, side dish, or soup.
  Canned beans are easy and fast. Look for low sodium or no salt added cans.
- 1-cup serving of beans has as much as 10 to 13 grams of fiber. Pair with a whole grain such as brown rice or quinoa.
- Have at least two vegetable servings at dinner. One-half cup cooked or 1 cup raw equals 1 serving.

OTHER SOURCES OF FIBER

- Snack bars (be sure to read the label)
- Kraft Foods line of 100% whole wheat crackers and cookies
- Flaxseed, chia seeds and bran can be added to yogurt and smoothies
- Mission or La Tortilla Factory whole grain tortilla wraps. Oher brands are available depending on the store.
- Fresh fruits and vegetables are portable snacks. Try throwing in a few pieces of fruit, individual packages of raisins or cranberries, or some baby carrots in your briefcase or backpack.
- Benefiber® provides a natural source of soluble fiber that can help with bowel issues. Each serving provides 3 grams of fiber and can be mixed into beverages or soft foods. Try adding it to water, pudding, milk, cereal, yogurt, pasta sauce, or gelatin.
- Metamucil crackers also provide a natural source of fiber and help maintain digestive health. Each serving contains 2 – 3 grams soluble fiber.

Source: Mayo Clinic, USDA National Nutrient Database.

Be aware that increasing your fiber intake too quickly can cause gas, diarrhea, and bloating. Increase your fiber intake gradually. Begin by adding about 5 grams of fiber each week. Increase your water intake as you increase fiber because fiber can also cause constipation, or "binding" of fiber in the colon. Adding more fiber to your daily diet is a wise investment in your health.

HOW MUCH FIBER IS IN THE FOOD I EAT?

Check the fiber food list below to see if you are getting 25-35 gram daily.

FRUITS

Food Item	Serving Size	Fiber Content
Apple	1 medium	3.3 g
Apricots, dried	8 halves	1g
Banana	1 medium	3.1 g
Blackberries	1/2 cup	4g
Blueberries	1 cup	3.5 g
Cantaloupe	1 wedge	0.6 g
Figs	2 medium	3.7 g
Grapes	1 cup	1.4 g
Kiwifruit	1 fruit	2.3 g
Orange	1 medium	3.1 g
Papaya	1 cup	2.5 g
Peach	1 medium	2.2 g
Pear	1 medium	5.1 g
Prunes	5 items	3g
Raspberries	1/2 cup	4g
Strawberries	1 cup	3.3 g
Tomato	1 medium	1.5 g
Watermelon	1 wedge	1.1 g

VEGETABLES

Food Item	Serving Size	Fiber Content
Artichoke	1/2cup	4.5g
Asparagus,cooked	1/2cup	1.8g

Bakedpotatow/skin	1medium	4.4g
Bakedsweetpotato	1medium	3.8g
Broccoli,raw	1cup	2.4g
BrusselsSprouts,cooked	1/2cup	2g
Cabbage,cooked	1cup	3g
Carrots	1medium	2g
Cauliflower,raw	1/2cup	1.2g
Celery,raw	1cup	1.6g
Collardgreens	1cup	1.5g
Corn	1cup	3.2g
Cucumbers	10slices	0.7g
Greenbeans,raw	1cup	3.7g
Jicama,raw	1/2cup	2.9g
Peas	1cup	8.8g
Redbellpepper,raw	1small	1.6g
Romainelettuce	1cup	1g
Turnipgreens	1/2cup	2.5g
Wintersquash,cooked	1cup	5.7g

LENTILS, BEANS AND NUTS		
Food Item	Serving Size	Fiber Content
Almonds	1 ounce	3.3 g
Baked beans	1 cup	16g
Black beans	1 cup	15g
Black-eyed peas	1/2 cup	3g
Cashews	1 ounce	0.9 g
Chickpeas	1/2 cup	5.3 g
Great northern beans	1/2 cup	7g

Kidney beans	1/2 cup	6.5 g
Lentils	1 cup	15.6 g
Lima Beans	1/2 cup	7g
Navy beans	1/2 cup	9g
Peanuts	1 ounce	2.4 g
Peas, split (green)	1 cup	8g
Pinto beans	1/2 cup	7.3 g
Pistachios	1 ounce	2.9 g
Soybeans (green)	1/2 cup	5g

GRAINS, CEREALS AND PASTAS		
Food Item	**Serving Size**	**Fiber Content**
All-Bran	1/2 cup	6.6 g
Barley, pearled	1 cup	6g
Brown rice	1 cup	3.5 g
Buckwheat, Soba Noodles	2 ounces	3g
Bulgur	1 cup	8g
Cheerios	1 cup	3g
Grape Nuts	1/2 cup	5g
Oatmeal, rolled	1/2 cup	5g
Quinoa	1 cup	4g
Raisin Bran	3/4 cup	3g
Shredded Wheat	1/2 cup	4g
White rice	1 cup	0.6 g
Whole wheat bread	1 slice	2g
Whole wheat spaghetti	1 cup	6.3 g

10 REASONS DRY BEANS PROMOTE HEART HEALTH

- Dry beans contain no sodium.
- Dry beans are a rich source of potassium.
- Dry beans contain no cholesterol.
- Dry beans are a fat-free food.
- Dry beans are a rich source of dietary fiber, including cholesterol-binding soluble fiber.
- Dry beans contain heart-healthy vegetable protein,
- Dry beans are an excellent source of folic acid.
- Dry bean consumption may help weight management
- People with diabetes who consume cooked, dry beans have a lower risk of heart disease.
- Dry beans pair well with other heart-healthy food like fish and olive oil.

Maureen Murtaugh, PhD, RD, "Dry Bean Quarterly" www.beaninstitute.com

OUR PICK FOR THE TOP 10 BEANS	
Black Beans	Excellent source of fiber, folate, iron, and magnesium
Black-Eyed Peas	Good source of fiber, magnesium, and zinc
Chickpea or Garbanzo Beans	High in fiber and folate and provide potassium and magnesium
Fava Beans	Excellent source of fiber and folate and provide iron, magnesium, and potassium
Great Northern Beans	Excellent source of fiber and folate
Kidney Beans	High in fiber and folate
Lima Beans	High in fiber and potassium

Navy Beans	High in folate and fiber
Red Beans	Excellent source of fiber and iron
Soybeans	Excellent source calcium, iron, potassium and nine essential amino acids

Answers to Fiber Questions

1. True
2. True
3. True
4. False-High fiber foods can make you feel full and aid in weight loss efforts.
5. False-Women should eat 25 grams fiber daily and men 38 grams

CALCIUM: ALLOWS US TO STAND

"Use the right ingredients and choose foods that are good for the bones, your body, and your soul, bon appétit."

— *Knute Rockne*

Calcium Questions: Test your knowledge by answering True or False to the questions below.

1. Men should not be concerned about calcium intake because they rarely have problems with bone density.
2. Consuming one glass of milk and one container of yogurt each day provides me with adequate calcium.
3. Calcium supplements should be taken between meals.
4. Osteoporosis is not a major issue in the United States.
5. Most of the calcium found in the body is stored in bones.
6. The most important dietary source of vitamin D is cheese.

Whether you're five, fifteen, or fifty, getting enough calcium in your diet is important. Adequate calcium intake can be a major concern for people who are always on the go because dairy products require refrigeration and are often unavailable. Yet new research has shown that individuals who consume adequate calcium are more likely to maintain a normal body weight. When you are running errands, picking up kids, or traveling for business, getting your daily requirement of calcium may take a little more effort than some of the other nutrients.

CALCIUM AND VITAMIN D

Before 18 years of age, our bone density has already been determined. The National Osteoporosis Foundation states that by our mid-thirties bones slowly begin to lose their mass. After that time, our bodies need calcium to replenish calcium stores. While dairy products are the best sources of calcium, vitamin D plays a vital role in the absorption of calcium. Milk fortified with vitamin D is the most important source of calcium in our diet. Cheese and yogurt are a good source of calcium, but they are not always fortified with vitamin D. Check your cheeses and yogurts to make sure they are fortified since many brands are now fortified with vitamin D.

VITAMIN D FOOD SOURCES INCLUDE:

- Fortified Milk
- Fortified Orange Juice
- Egg yolk
- Fish Liver Oils
- Fortified Margarines
- Herring
- Fortified Butters
- Salmon
- Fortified Cereals
- Mushrooms grown in UV light
- Some yogurts and cheese

Vitamin D can also be obtained from sunlight. Fifteen minutes in direct sun, without sun block, can provide your daily vitamin D requirement. In colder climates, the amount of vitamin D received from the sun is minimal so it is crucial to insure adequate dietary intake.

FACTORS THAT CAN REDUCE THE AMOUNT OF VITAMIN D OBTAINED FROM SUNLIGHT:

- Age
- Season
- Glass windows with UV protection
- Sunscreen use
- Latitude
- Clothing (especially covering the forearms)

VITAMIN D BENEFITS

- Reduces inflammation
- Regulates mental health
- Aids in synthesis of serotonin and dopamine
- Helps in immune building
- Helps increase the levels of glutathione in the body necessary for natural detoxification

There has been concern recently about the incidence of vitamin D deficiency. The National Health and Nutrition Examination Survey (NHANES) showed that few race, age, or gender groups meet the current dietary intake recommendations for vitamin D. It is estimated that 50% of the adult population is vitamin D deficient.

Vitamin D Deficiency Has Been Associated With

- Increased risk of heart disease
- Bone and muscle weakness
- High blood pressure
- Congestive heart failure
- Chronic blood vessel inflammation associated with hardening of the arteries
- Certain cancers
- Multiple sclerosis
- Increased risk of Type1 Diabetes in offspring of mothers with low Vitamin D intakes in pregnancy
- Potential for increasing Type1 Diabetes in children genetically susceptible to the condition

Vitamin D DRIs from the Food and Nutrition Board of the Institute of Medicine 2011	
Age group	**Dietary Reference Intake**
Infants 0-6 months	400 IU (10 mcg)
Infants 7-12 months	400 IU (10 mcg)
Children 1-3 years	600 IU (15 mcg)
Children 4-8 years	600 IU (15 mcg)
Children and Adults 9-70 years	600 IU (15 mcg)
Adults > 70 years	800 IU (20 mcg)
Pregnancy & Lactation	600 IU (15 mcg)

Calcium Recommendations from the Food and Nutrition Board of the Institute of Medicine 2011	
Age group	Dietary Reference Index
Infants 0-6 months	200 mg
Infants 7-12 months	260 mg
Children 1-3 years	700 mg
Children 4-8 years	1000 mg
Children 9-18 years	1300 mg
Adults 19-50 years	1000 mg
Adults 51-70 years (Male)	1000 mg
Adults 51-70 years (Female)	1200 mg
Adults 71+ years	1200 mg
Postmenopausal or any amenorrhoeic woman who is taking estrogen	1000 mg
Postmenopausal or any amenorrhoeic woman who is not taking estrogen	1500 mg
Pregnant or breastfeeding women 14-18 years	1300 mg
Pregnant or breastfeeding women >19 years	1000 mg

WHY DOES THE BODY REQUIRE CALCIUM AND VITAMIN D?

Bone is constantly in the process of building and breaking down. When bones break down, the bone cells called osteoclasts dissolve old bone. When bones begin to rebuild, bone cells called osteoblasts pull calcium and other minerals from the blood. These minerals, together with the structural protein, collagen, reforms bone tissue. The osteoclasts and osteoblasts are always in balance until the age of 30 when the balance begins to change. At this time the bones begin to break down faster and women, in particular, lose more bone than they are making. This loss further accelerates after menopause when estrogen levels fall. Estrogen works to regulate the activity of the osteoclasts, or cells that breakdown bone causing a significant increase in the incidence of osteoporosis. It has been estimated that 7.4 million women over the age of 50 have osteoporosis. The blood also maintains a constant level of calcium and if it is unable to do so, the body takes it from bone. Vitamin D deficiency can also lead to brittle bones because vitamin D aids in the absorption of calcium.

Warding off osteoporosis is crucial in preventing bone fractures and their possible deadly consequences. It has been estimated that for a year after a hip fracture, women over age 65 are twice as likely to die, as they would be with no fracture.

Fewer than 25% of women are estimated to get their necessary calcium and vitamin D from food and most do not get enough vitamin D from sunlight to prevent vitamin D deficiency. Approximately 42% of Americans are deficient and deficiency is common in cold climates where exposure to sunlight is minimal. This is why medical experts urge the use of calcium and vitamin D supplements.

FACTS ABOUT CALCIUM

- The body gets the calcium it needs from the diet or takes what it needs from bones.
- Calcium is the most abundant mineral in the body; it is used to make bones and keep them strong.
- Ninety-nine percent of the calcium in the body is stored in the bones and teeth. The remainder of the body's calcium circulates in the blood and body tissues.
- Circulating calcium allows for muscle contraction, nerve conduction, blood clotting, iron utilization, activation of enzymes for metabolism, and regulation of nutrients in and out of cell walls.

- If there is not enough calcium in the blood and tissues, the body takes calcium from the bones to meet its needs. When this happens, the bones lose their strength and often break.

- During menopause and periods of amenorrhea, bone loss is accelerated due to the lack of the hormone estrogen, which affects the absorption of calcium. Adequate dietary intake of calcium can reduce the risk of bone loss.

IMPORTANT CONCERNS ABOUT CALCIUM ABSORBTION

Recent research suggests that drinking colas and other soft drinks may be bad for your bones. The American Journal of Clinical Nutrition reported the results of studies showing an association between soft drink intake and lower bone mineral density regardless of age, menopause, and calcium and vitamin D intake. When substituting soft drinks for milk, calcium and vitamin D intake can be compromised. Additionally, excessive caffeine consumption is linked to a higher risk of osteoporosis.

Calcium Recommendations from the Food and Nutrition Board of the Institute of Medicine 2011	
Fiber	Adequate fiber intake is vital to keeping the digestive tract moving, reducing constipation, and decreasing the chance of diverticulosis (the formation of small pouches in the lining of the colon usually due to low fiber intake). However, large amounts of fiber, in particular bran, can decrease calcium absorption.
Protein	Adequate protein intake is crucial in calcium absorption, but excessive protein intake can increase urinary calcium excretion.

Meal Time	Some calcium supplements need to be taken with meals. This will ensure adequate calcium absorption by allowing stomach acids to dissolve and absorb the calcium. Be sure to read the supplement label for directions.
Caffeine	Drinking more than four cups of caffeinated coffee a day can increase calcium excretion. Also, soft drinks with caffeine can cause calcium loss.
Sodium	Excessive sodium consumption can increase urinary calcium.
Green Leafy Vegetables	Oxalates and oxalic acid (found in green leafy vegetables) bind with calcium during digestion, making calcium insoluble. Calcium DRI's take this into account and a mixed diet minimizes this issue.

Studies have also shown that a diet high in sodium can rob the body of calcium. Other studies have shown that the lack of potassium and magnesium can be the culprits in reducing the body's supply of calcium. Dairy products are not only high in calcium, but also contain high levels of magnesium and potassium.

The acid-base balance of the diet and its effect on bone and muscle health is an area that is being researched. Acid load contributed by the diet is not handled well by the elderly due to reduction in kidney function. The increase in acid concentration in the bloodstream causes muscle wasting because muscle and bone loss is the body's adaptation to excess acid. Grain products (bread, cereal, crackers, rice, and dessert items) increase acid levels. Fruits and vegetables are broken down to bicarbonate and add alkali to the body that neutralizes acid.

Another area of concern for risk of hip fracture is too much vitamin A retinol. Some research studies have found that very high doses of vitamin A can lead to massive bone loss and coma. To avoid this potential risk, vitamin A should be limited to 2000 to 3000 IU of retinol each day.

Osteoporosis is a condition that is characterized by a decrease of bone mass and bone density. The United States has one of the highest rates of osteoporosis in the world, with 15-20 million people affected and 80% of those people are women. Although osteoporosis is generally associated with post-menopausal women, over 2 million men also have been diagnosed with osteoporosis, and over 3 million men are at risk. It has been estimated that one out of eight men over the age of 50 will break a bone due to osteoporosis. The American Geriatric Society states that 20 to 24% of people who experience a hip fracture will die within the first year after the fracture. Adequate calcium intake is critically important to minimize these changes. (Check the Exercise Chapter for information on resistance and strength training exercises that help to enhance bone density.)

Risk factors that place you at higher risk of osteoporosis		
Uncontrollable	**Controllable**	**Secondary Risks**
Female (although males can get it also)	Diet low in calcium and vitamin D	Cancer
Postmenopausal	Cigarette smoking	Rheumatoid arthritis
Family history of osteoporosis	Excessive alcohol use	Men with low testosterone levels
Advanced Age Caucasian or Asian	Inactivity	Blood thinners Use of Anti-depressants
Slender body build		Prior bariatric surgery for weight loss
Early Menopause		Diabetes

Delayed Periods	Eating disorder
	Use of anti-depressants
	Use of glucocorticoids for several months (for instance, prednisone
	Hormonal treatments to prevent reoccurrence of breast/ prostate cancer

*Adequate vitamin D is needed for calcium absorption as well as muscle synthesis. It increases lower back strength, decreases body sway, and helps with instability to reduce falls that can result in fractures. Because it is fat soluble, take with your largest meal containing fat.

SIX OTHER BONE-BUILDING FOOD HELPERS

- Fish is an important addition to a bone-building diet due to its vitamin D content that helps absorb calcium. The best fish is salmon. A 3-½ ounce serving will provide almost 90% of your daily vitamin D requirement.

- Seeds are an important source of magnesium that is found in healthy bones. Fifty percent of our body's magnesium is found in bones. All seeds provide magnesium, but pumpkin seeds are the highest source.

- Beans especially black, white, and kidney beans are high in magnesium and calcium. The US Dietary Guidelines for Americans recommends a weekly intake of 2 ½ cups of beans and other legumes. These would include peas and legumes.

- Nuts, especially walnuts, contain a rich source of alpha linolenic acid, an omega-3 fatty acid that helps in the reduction of bone breakdown and aids in bone formation.

- Leafy greens supply bone-building calcium, magnesium, and vitamin K. Vitamin K is crucial in the building of bones because they form bone proteins and cut calcium loss in the urine.

- Oysters contain our best source of zinc in the diet. Zinc helps in the formation of bone collagen that forms the protein framework of bones that allows them to be flexible.

DIETARY CALCIUM SOURCES

Good dietary sources of calcium include milk, yogurt, and cheese. Other non-dairy sources include tofu, sardines and salmon (with bones), almonds, broccoli, and collard greens. The charts that follow will show you some common sources of dietary calcium. Look on the label of most prepared products to find the % Daily Value calcium need based upon a 2,000-calorie diet. When reading the label, check the label for the % Daily Value for calcium. If a food has 40% calcium, it contains 400 mg calcium (remove the % sign and add a zero).

1000 mg Calcium
- 1 cup General Mills Raisin Bran Total cereal
- ¾ cup General Mill Whole Grain Total cereal
- 1 1/3 cup Total Corn Flakes cereal
- 1 ¼ cup Harmony cereal * 600 mg

500 mg Calcium
- 1 cup Lactaid Calcium-fortified milk
- 1 packet Quaker Oatmeal Nutrition for Women

300 - 500 mg Calcium
- 1 cup skim, 2 %, or whole milk
- 1 cup plain yogurt
- 1 cup orange juice fortified with calcium
- 1 cup cereal with 30% calcium
- 1 Sports bar with 30% calcium

- 1 cup Soy milk fortified with calcium (varies)
- ½ cup calcium enriched tofu
- 1 Starbucks Fat-free Tall Latte
- 1-ounce Kraft 2% grated cheddar cheese * 400 mg
- Krusteaz Fat-Free Calcium Enriched Muffins
- 1 cup Ronzoni Smart Taste Pasta

200 - 300 mg Calcium

- 1 oz. most cheeses
- 1 slice calcium-enriched bread
- 1 cup 1% or 2% chocolate milk
- 1 cup macaroni and cheese
- 1 large slice cheese pizza
- Fortified Cereal or Granola Bars (varies)
- Instant Breakfast drink
- Crystal-lite powdered drink mix enriched with Calcium

Minimum of 100 mg Calcium

- ½ cup broccoli
- ½ cup pudding
- 1 oz. Ricotta cheese
- 1 cup light ice cream or regular ice cream
- ½ cup tofu made with calcium sulfate
- 3 oz. Canned salmon with bones
- ½ cup cooked collards
- 1 tbs. Blackstrap molasses
- 1 cup Cheerios (regular, Team, Frosted, Honey)
- 1 cup cereal with 10% calcium
- 2 Kellogg's Eggo Waffles
- 1 can 7up Plus berry soda
- 1 cup kale

Diets rich in dairy foods have been shown to reduce the prevalence of metabolic syndrome in obese individuals. A prospective study of obese individuals in Caerphilly, UK, found men who regularly drank a pint of milk or more daily had reduced their odds of developing metabolic syndrome by 21%.

There has been a trend towards taking both a calcium and vitamin D supplement to ward off osteoporosis. In 2012, Americans spent $1.2 billion on calcium supplements and $652 million on vitamin D pills.

In 2013, the U.S. Preventive Services Task Force studied over 16 randomized, controlled studies and concluded that daily supplements of calcium and vitamin D do not protect healthy postmenopausal women from fractures and should not be recommended. It also concluded that the supplements did not help pre- menopausal women either.

Two British studies done in 2005 concluded that calcium pills, even with vitamin D did not prevent fractures. In 2006, the Women's Health Initiative found that women taking 1000 mg of calcium and 400 mg of vitamin D for 7 years are no less likely to experience a hip injury.

The British Medical Journal reported that the use of calcium supplements needs to be reconsidered. This is due to a number of studies that showed the use of calcium supplements either with or without Vitamin D showed an increase in heart attacks. Dr. Mark J. Boland of the University of Auckland in New Zealand also questions the use of calcium supplements since they reduce fracture risk only marginally.

There are many osteoporosis experts and the National Osteoporosis Foundation who are not ready to tell Americans to stop supplementation. Since the body cannot make calcium and vitamin D synthesis requires sunlight, most nutritionists and osteoporosis experts still tell patients to attempt to meet requirements with food and exposure to sunlight without sunscreen. If this is not possible, supplementation is suggested. Calcium need should be determined after finding your individual requirement, finding what your usual calcium intake is, and adding the necessary amount needed from supplements.

Another interesting study was reported by Dr. Peter Schnatz from the Reading Hospital and Medical Center in West Reading, Pa. He reported in the Journal Menopause that supplementation of both calcium and vitamin D could help improve women's cholesterol levels.

Calcium intake can be compromised by lactose intolerance. Nutrition Today (Sept. 2009) suggests that the prevalence of lactose intolerance may be lower than previously believed. If you feel lactose in milk causes you problems, try the:

National Dairy Council's tips to minimize problems with milk products:

D	Drink milk with meals
A	Aged cheeses like cheddar and Swiss are low in lactose
I	Introduce dairy slowly, gradually increase the amount consumed
R	Reduce lactose by enjoying lactose-free milk and milk products
Y	Yogurt with active cultures helps to digest lactose

Lactose intolerance can be helped by the use of Dairy Ease and Lactaid, and other over the counter products. These products contain the lactose enzyme that helps in digesting dairy products. Although helpful to some, not everyone is helped with these products. Symptoms of lactose intolerance include: indigestion, cramping, bloating, and diarrhea. A product that has gained popularity for those with lactose intolerance is Fairlife Ultra--filtered milk that has 50% more protein and 50% less sugar than milk. The company also produces ice cream, yogurt, creamer, and shakes.

Is refrigeration of dairy products causing you to avoid calcium? If so, try to meet your calcium needs with cheese on your sandwich, yogurt, or calcium-enriched food items. If you are unable to obtain low-fat yogurt and cheese when traveling or ordering lunch on the go, bring a calcium supplement with you to allow for your calcium needs while keeping your dietary intake lower in calories, fat, and cholesterol.

Calcium supplements come in a number of varieties	
Calcium Citrate	Calcium citrate is more readily absorbable. It can be taken at any time of the day and is not dependent on eating.
Calcium Gluconate and Calcium Lactate	Calcium gluconate and calcium lactate supplements contain less calcium per dose, making them costlier and less convenient.
Chelated Calcium	Chelated supplements are not absorbed any better than other supplements; therefore, the additional cost is not justifiable.
Calcium Phosphate	Calcium phosphate supplements should be avoided because the excess phosphorus could reduce calcium metabolism.
Oyster Shell	Oyster shell supplements should be avoided because they may contain toxic contaminants such as lead.
Cal-100 with D	Cal-100 with vitamin D provides 1000 mg of calcium and is found in a pre-measured, powdered form. Cal-100 is tasteless, non-gritty, and can be mixed with beverages or most solid foods. When mixed with orange juice, it produces a low acid, lightly carbonated beverage. This product is perfect for individuals who have problems swallowing large calcium tablets.

Calcium Carbonate	Calcium carbonate is the most common calcium supplement. It can be found in chewable, capsule, tablet, and antacid forms. Viactiv is a popular chew that supplies 500 mg calcium in each serving. Calcium carbonate needs to be taken twice a day at meals to meet the RDA for calcium. Be sure to take it with meals to ensure adequate calcium absorption by allowing stomach acid to be produced to dissolve and absorb the calcium.

Answers to Calcium Questions:

1. False. Men do need to worry about bone density. Over 2 million men have osteoporosis and over 3 million men are at risk in the United States.

2. False. Most people need more than a glass of milk and one container of yogurt each day to meet their calcium needs.

3. False. Most calcium supplements are best taken with meals. Calcium citrate does not need to be taken with meals.

4. False-Osteoporosis is a major health concern in the United States.

5. True

6. False. The most important dietary source of Vitamin D is milk.

PREBIOTICS AND PROBIOTICS: MAINTAINING GUT HEALTH

Probiotics are a fascinating topic that has gained much interest over the last several years. Research has shown positive effects on many conditions including Parkinson's disease, obesity, metabolic syndrome and cardiovascular disease as well as on the immune system. Companies that make probiotic foods and supplements promote these health benefits and more with far more certainty than the research supports.

Gut microbiota or gut flora and probiotics are not the same. The gut microbiota comprises friendly microorganisms in the intestinal tract -- mainly bacteria, yeast and viruses. Most are found in the large intestine or colon. These microorganism make vitamin K and some B vitamins. They also convert fiber into short-chain fatty acids. These fats feed the microbes but also stimulate the human immune system and support the walls of the GI tract.

The American College of Gastroenterology states that trillions of bacteria live in our digestive tract and more than 400 species have been identified. When the gut microbiome is disrupted, the immune system can be compromised, resulting in an increased risk of infection. Diet and medications such as antibiotics can also throw the gut microbiome into disarray. Research has shown diets high in fat can upset the delicate balance in the gut, which may play a role in the development of obesity, but a high fiber diet is beneficial.

The Food and Agriculture Organization of the United Nations and World Health Organization define probiotics as "live microorganisms which when administered in adequate amounts confer a health benefit on the host." They can enhance the immune system and promote intestinal health and regularity.

Probiotics are found in fermented foods that have live and active cultures. Some fermented foods that contain these bacteria are yogurt, soy drinks, miso, sauerkraut, and fermented and unfermented milk. When you read labels make sure it says "live and active" culture, e.g., lactobacillus. The most well-known probiotic species include lactobacillus, bifidobacterium, and saccharomyces. Probiotics can also be taken as supplements; none are approved or regulated as drugs.

Purported Benefits of Probiotic Supplements:

- Synthesize vitamins
- Boost the immune system
- Improve allergies, particularly related to the skin
- Decrease the risk of dental caries
- Speed recovery from bacterial vaginosis
- Decrease symptoms of inflammatory bowel disease
- Help those with lactose intolerance digest dairy products
- Reduce symptoms of diarrhea associated with antibiotics

Probiotic supplements are formulated to assure that the bacteria can survive the acidic environment of the stomach and colonize the small intestine and colon. Some can secrete chemicals that prevent toxins from breaking down.

BEFORE YOU BUY, CONSIDER:

1. Is the probiotic for a specific condition or general health. Different strains of probiotic are recommended for different conditions.

2. Not all probiotics are the same. There are hundreds of probiotic supplements available with a single strain to multiple strains. The effective dose depends on the strain.

3. The number of colony forming units identifies the number of viable microbes in a dose. A higher dose of probiotics does not increase the effect.

4. The American College of Gastroenterology Patient Education and Resource Center says there is no evidence to support the claim that either preparations with multiple species/strains or higher concentrations of bacteria leads to improved health.

5. Read the label and look for the health benefits, storage, and expiration date.

6. Supplements are not regulated or tested as stringently as prescription medications.

7. Price does not equal quality and effectiveness.

8. For overall health, try food first.

Research is limited on the benefits, but preliminary findings have shown positive benefits. Different strains work best for different health conditions. So, a probiotic that works well for managing antibiotic associated diarrhea may not be effective for managing inflammation or IBS symptoms. General side effects from taking probiotics include gas and bloating, especially in the first few weeks.

Prebiotics' role is to feed probiotic organisms, helping to increase the number in our digestive system. Prebiotics can be found in a variety of foods and are also available in supplements that include powder, capsules, tablets, and drops. The two most common prebiotics are inulin and oligofructose. Inulin is found in artichokes, asparagus, onions, garlic, bananas, wheat, rye, and chicory root. Oligofructose is found in fruits. Two other prebiotics are resistant starch and galacto-oligosaccharide. These starches are found naturally in raw potatoes, cooked and cooled starchy foods, and unripe bananas. They are also added to some packaged pasta, dairy and bakery items, cereals and cereal bars, and some table spreads. Companies don't have to tell you how much is in a product.

You can find more information by visiting these websites: International Food Information Council and International Scientific Association for Probiotics and Prebiotics: www.isapp.net and the International Food Information Council Foundation: www.foodinsight.org.

POSSIBLE PREBIOTIC BENEFITS

1. Maintain a healthy digestive system
2. Allow beneficial bacteria to grow instead of harmful bacteria
3. Strengthen the body's immune system
4. Improve bowel function
5. Increase mineral absorption of calcium, iron, and magnesium
6. Help lower cholesterol

FOODS CONTAINING PREBIOTICS

1. Chicory Root
2. Garlic
3. Jerusalem Artichoke
4. Leeks
5. Wheat

6. Legumes
7. Barley
8. Rye
9. Asparagus
10. Flax
11. Leafy Greens
12. Oatmeal
13. Onion
14. Bananas
15. Honey

The following organizations can provide more information about Probiotics

- American Gastroenterological Association
- American College of Gastroenterology
- Academy of Nutrition and Dietetics
- National Center for Complementary and Alternative Medicine
- American Academy of Microbiology
- International Scientific Association for Probiotics and Prebiotics
- World Gastroenterology Organization
- Food and Agriculture Organization of the United Nations/ World Health Organization

SUPER FOODS

"I'm strong to the finish when I eats my spinach"

— Popeye

A super food conjures up a vision of Popeye developing super strength after eating spinach. The popular media has grasped on to this idea with more than 40 items being identified as "super foods". Super foods are known for high nutrient content and are called nutrient dense. We like to call them " celebrity foods". Like some celebrities, they may be popular for a while only to be replaced with another in due time. More often than not, they are vegetables or fruits but can include other foods like nuts, seeds, grains, etc. The problem with eating excessive amounts of one nutrient dense food is that you might miss out on other healthy foods and their nutritional benefits.

The juicing craze especially "green juicing" usually includes large amounts of kale, broccoli, kassala, or bok choy. These contain a chemical called thiocyanate, making it goitrogenic. Goitrogens are substances that interfere with the uptake of iodine and cause an enlargement of the thyroid gland in people with thyroid disease. Large amounts of fat-soluble vitamins vitamin A and K can also be found in these foods and can be toxic to the body.

We can't help but preach that "more is not necessarily better" when it comes to these assumed super foods. Many foods get far more attention than they deserve and may wind up causing serious health consequences.

The Academy of Nutrition and Dietetics (AND) stresses that although there are foods that are high in certain nutrients, phytochemicals, and antioxidants, it is important to eat a "super diet". This means following the Dietary Guidelines for Americans covered in our book. These guidelines along with consuming "super foods", exercising regularly, and practicing healthy behaviors will help improve your health and reduce disease. You will find the chart below that highlights foods that supply good nutrition, but AND's guidelines should be kept in mind.

Asparagus	Nutrients: Highest folic acid of any vegetable and one of the most nutritionally balanced. High in fiber, rich in Vitamin A
	Health Benefits: Protects against cancer, colon in particular, enhances heart health, increases immunity
Beans, Legumes	Nutrients: High Fiber, protein, vitamins, minerals, phyto- nutrients
	Health Benefit: Enhances heart health, reduces colon cancer, smoothes blood sugars
Blueberries	Nutrients: High fiber, high in anti-oxidants
	Health Benefits: Enhances heart health, protects body against disease, promotes immunity, slows age-related brain decline, smoothes blood sugars
Broccoli	Nutrients: Considered one of the healthiest vegetables and is called a triple super food. Provides 10% of the daily requirement of iron. One of the highest vegetable sources of calcium. Rich source of fiber and vitamin A
	Health Benefits: Enhances heart health, reduces colon cancer, smoothes blood sugars, promotes healthy bones and teeth, and promotes immune function

Collard Greens	Nutrients: Rich source of vitamin A, vitamin C, and vitamin K. Contains phytochemicals such as carotenoids and flavonoids. High in fiber
	Health Benefits: Enhances heart health, promotes immunity, smoothes blood sugars, protects against cancer, and promotes healthy bones and teeth
Dark Chocolate	Nutrients: Packed with antioxidants
	Health Benefit: Preliminary research shows it may lower blood pressure
Green Peas	Nutrients: One of the highest vegetable sources of protein. Rich source of fiber, vitamin A. Considered a vitamin powerhouse
	Health Benefits: Protects against colon cancer, increases immunity, promotes healthy bones and teeth, enhances heart health
Kale	Nutrients: Rich source of vitamin A, vitamin C, vitamin K, and fiber. Contains phytochemicals such as carotenoids and flavonoids
	Health Benefits: Protects against colon cancer, increases immunity, promotes healthy bones and teeth, enhances heart health
Kiwi	Nutrients: Most nutrient dense popular fruit. Contains more vitamin C than oranges in equal amounts
	Health Benefits: Increases immune function, enhances heart health, decreases colon cancer
Oranges	Nutrients: High source of vitamin C, high fiber, and cancer-fighting phytochemicals. Heath Benefits: Enhances heart health, increases immune function, promotes healthy skin and eyes, and protects against cancer

Papaya	Nutrients: Rich source of vitamin C and fiber. Health Benefits: Promotes healthy skin and heart health. Enhances immune function, smoothes blood sugars, and decreases colon cancer risk
Pumpkin	Nutrients: Highest fruit or vegetable source of vitamin A. High in fiber. Health Benefits: Promotes healthy skin and eyes. Enhances heart health, increases immune function, and decreases colon cancer risk
Salmon	Nutrients: High in Omega-3 fatty acids. Heath Benefits: Enhances heart health, reduces arthritis symptoms, and may help depression
Strawberries	Nutrients: High in antioxidants, vitamin C, and phytonutrients. Health Benefits: Enhances heart health, increases good cholesterol, lowers blood pressure, protects against cancer, and reduces inflammation
Tea (Green or Black)	Nutrients: Contains potent antioxidants and flavonoids that are related to decreased incidence of stroke and build-up of plaque in the arteries. Benefits: Tea is the most consumed beverage in the world with less caffeine than coffee and zero calories. *Green tea is lower in caffeine and higher in flavonoids than black tea. *Herbal teas like chamomile have been found to reduce stress and increase comfort. Tea's intake has increased during Covid19 possibly due to these benefits
Tomatoes	Nutrients: Contains the cancer-fighting antioxidant lycopene. Health Benefits: Prevents many types of cancer

Turkey	Nutrients: One of leanest animal proteins. Contains the amino acid tryptophan. High in folic acid. Health Benefits: Protects against birth defects, some cancers, and heart disease with its folic acid content. Tryptophan content helps to reduce moodiness, helps with sleep, promotes calmness, and stimulates the immune system
Walnuts	Nutrients: High source of fiber, polyphenols, vitamin E, magnesium, and vitamin B6. Health Benefits: Enhances heart health and decreases chance of diabetes and cancer
Yogurt	Contains probiotics that preliminary research suggest may help with digestive disorders, bacterial and yeast infections, food allergies, and immune function.

SUGAR: A HIDDEN DANGER?

The dangers of too much added sugar has taken root in social media and online in recent years. And so has some of the misconceptions and inaccuracies about different types of sugars and added sugars.

The sugar most think about is white sugar and brown sugar. But sugar occurs naturally in foods as well, such as fruit (fructose and glucose) and milk (lactose). Sugars or syrups are added to food during processing and preparation is what we should really be focused on reducing. But beware: Added sugars go by many names. These include brown sugar, corn sweeteners, corn syrup, dextrose, fructose, glucose, high-fructose corn syrup, agave, honey, lactose, malt syrup, maltose, molasses, maple syrup, raw sugar, and sucrose. Yes, even the "natural sugars" honey, agave and maple syrup still count as added sugar.

Consuming too much sugar can lead to feelings of depression, anxiety, and jitteriness. When we eat foods that are high in sugar, our blood sugar rises rapidly and then drops swiftly, which sparks these reactions in our body and brain. Too much sugar can also increase the risk of dental cavities, worsening joint pain, and inflammation which can increase our risk for some chronic diseases.

Those chronic diseases include non-alcoholic fatty liver disease (NAFLD) and non-alcoholic steatohepatitis (NASH), which can result in scarring of the liver and long-term damage. The scarring cuts off the blood supply to the liver causing cirrhosis and the need for a liver transplant. Inflammation also occurs in the heart causing artery walls to thicken and permanent damage. The result is the increased risk of heart failure, heart attacks, and strokes.

Consuming less added sugar has been found to reduce those spikes in blood sugar and a lower average blood sugar. Large spikes in blood sugar and a rising average blood sugar means the pancreas must work extra hard to produce enough insulin to lower our blood sugar. Plus lots of foods high in sugar increases the risk of added weight and inflammation, which impairs the body's ability to use the insulin it does produce. Together that increases the risk of diabetes. The kidneys are also affected when the body cannot handle sugar causing kidney damage over time.

Average Americans consume an average of about 17 teaspoons of added sugar daily or approximately 57 pounds of added sugar each year. The American Heart Association recommends reducing this amount to 9 teaspoons of sugar for men daily and 6 teaspoons of sugar for woman. Current research shows that 77% of Americans have reduced their intake of sugar in recent years. The biggest change has come from a drop in regular soda. A 12 oz serving of regular soda contains about 8 teaspoons (32 grams) of added sugar and 128 calories. Americans are also being urged to cut back even more on sugar by a Federal Committee. This scientific group is concerned with the numerous health risks caused by excessive sugar use. They are urging Americans to reduce their consumption of sugar to 10% of daily calories. For a diet of 2000 calories this would amount to 200 calories from sugar daily or the equivalent of 10 teaspoons of sugar.

A food's sugar content is important when selecting foods. Check the Nutrition Facts Label for the *total carbohydrate* content. Under this heading look for sugar. This is how much sugar (in grams) that is in one serving of your food. Every 4 grams of sugar on the label is the equivalent to adding a teaspoon of sugar to the food. If a food label states it contains 14 grams of sugar that is the equivalent of 3 ½ teaspoons of sugar.

When you are selecting foods, keep the following in mind:

- Choose breakfast cereals that contain less than 6 grams of sugar
- Look for yogurts that contain less than 10 grams of sugar. Lactose is responsible for some of this sugar so read the ingredient list
- Limit sodas, cakes, cookies, candy and ice cream the most common sources of added sugar and select fruit for dessert
- Avoid sweetened beverages and fruit juices and discover no sugar added beverages that you enjoy. Try flavoring your water with lemons or limes or a favorite fresh fruit.

It is important to remember that a little sugar is OK. A good rule of thumb is to save 10% of your calories for sugar added foods. If your caloric need is 2000 calories, consuming 200 calories from dessert items should not cause a problem. Monica and I have found with our children and grandchildren that it is more prudent to allow occasional sweets rather than prohibiting them. When particular foods are not permitted, it can increase the desire for them. And keep in mind that sweets should be viewed as "treats" not cheats.

SWEETENERS: Other Types of Sugar

Pink, blue, yellow, green and more. Pick your packet. Sugar substitutes or artificial sweeteners have been around for decades, and more are seeking a place on shelves and tables. Sugar substitutes add sweetness without the calories and improve the flavor and texture of foods. Some sugar substitutes have no influence on blood glucose levels, or they may have a small effect.

There have been some false claims that sugar substitutes can increase a person's craving for sweets. There is no scientific evidence to support this claim, and the sweeteners on the market have been tested and deemed safe.

There are two types of sugar substitutes: non-nutritive, containing no calories, and nutritive sweeteners, which do contain calories. They have all been tested and proved safe for people up to the Acceptable Daily Intake (ADI). The ADI is determined by a review of all available safety and toxicological data on a food additive. It is given as milligrams per kilogram body weight (mg/kg). Most consumers would have a difficult time reaching an intake as high as the ADIs.

Nonnutritive sweeteners include: Acesulfame Potassium (Ace-K), Aspartame, Neotame, Saccharin, Sucralose, and Stevia. They do not cause dental cavities and have no effect on blood glucose, cholesterol, or triglyceride levels.

- **Ace-K** is 200 times sweeter than sugar. It can withstand high temperatures used in cooking and baking. The human body does not metabolize Ace-K and excretes it through the urine unchanged. Ace-K's ADI is 15 mg/kg body weight. It is found in over 4,000 food products and is marketed with the names Sunett and Sweet One.

- **Aspartame** has been used as a tabletop sweetener since 1981 and has been added to foods and beverages since 1996. Aspartame is 200 times sweeter than sugar. It is absorbed into the bloodstream and used in normal body functions. People with phenylketonuria (PKU), a rare metabolic hereditary disease, should not use aspartame. It has been extensively researched and is considered safe for everyone else. Through the years, individuals have complained of physical issues from using aspartame, including headaches, dizziness, and seizures. But these claims have never been substantiated by research. Aspartame is found in hot and cold beverages, cereals, gelatins, puddings, ice cream, yogurt, candy, gum, and pharmaceuticals. Aspartame can be used in recipes, but when cooked for long periods of time, it loses its sweetness. Equal (blue packet) is the most common brand.

- **Neotame** is similar to aspartame but sweeter -- approximately 7,000-13,000 times sweeter than aspartame. It is partially absorbed by the small intestine and is rapidly metabolized. Only 20% of the phenylalanine is absorbed in the bloodstream so it is safe for people with PKU. Neotame can be used in baking, but with its intensive sweetness, it is usually blended with sugar first. It is not as widely used or as available as other nonnutritive sweeteners.

- **Saccharin** is the oldest approved sweetener and is 300 times sweeter than sugar. It has been used for over a century, and more than 30 studies have supported its safety. In 2000, the National Toxicology Program eliminated saccharin from its list of carcinogens. Sweet n Low (pink packet) is the most common brand.

- **Sucralose,** approved by the FDA in 1999, is 600 times sweeter than sugar. It is also heat-stable so it can be used for cooking. Over 20 years of research and testing have determined that sucralose is a safe product. Splenda (yellow packet) is the most common brand.

- **Stevia** is made from a plant that is related to chrysanthemums and ragweed. The sweetener, which is 200 times sweeter than sugar, is made from an extract of stevia leaf called rebaudioside A (Reb-A). Japanese companies have been producing sweeteners extracted from this South American plant for decades. Brands include Truvia, Zing, SweetLeaf, Stevia in the Raw, Pyure, and others. Splenda also has a stevia-based sweetener. The packets are usually green, green and white, or purple.

- **Polyols** are reduced-calorie sweeteners. They are not sugars or alcohols, but they have a similar chemical structure to both. They are low-digestible carbohydrates that contain half the calories of sugar and provide fewer calories per gram than other carbohydrates. Polyols taste like sugar and have a similar texture. They add bulk to products and a smooth texture to ice cream, fillings, frosting, yogurt, and fruit spreads. Polyols help with good oral health by decreasing tooth demineralization and dental caries as well as neutralizing plaque. They are also helpful in weight loss and weight maintenance and reduce overall glycemic load.

When calculating the total carbohydrate from a food sweetened totally from polyols, food with less than 10 grams of carbohydrate is considered a "free food". With greater than 10 grams of carbohydrate in a food, subtract half of the polyol grams from the total carbohydrates and then calculate the exchanges. Consuming more than 50 grams of polyols can cause GI upset. These symptoms are usually mild and temporary. Individuals will generally adapt in a few days.

- Xylitol is a sugar alcohol that has a mild artificial flavor. Cakes made with it are moist. Consumed in large amounts, it can cause diarrhea, bloating, or gas in some people.

  Often sweeteners are used in combination to improve taste, texture, reduce calories and increase the shelf life of foods. Consumers have also found that varying their use of sweeteners allows them to improve the taste and stability of products.

- Alitame is a new sweetener that Pfizer is seeking approval for use in the U.S. It is 2,000 times sweeter than sugar and has good heat stability. Cyclamate reapproval is also being sought, although it is presently approved in over 50 countries. It is 30 times sweeter than sugar and when used with other sweeteners is acceptable.

The following chart is an example from www.caloriecontrol. org, that describes the approximate number of servings of different aspartame-containing products that an adult and child would need to consume to reach the ADI of 50mg/kg of body weight.

Aspartame-Containing Product	Approximate number of servings per day to reach the ADI	
	Adult (150 lb.)	Child (50 lb.)
Carbonated Soft Drink (12 oz)	20	6
Powdered Soft Drink (8 oz)	30	11
Gelatin (4 oz)	42	14
Tabletop Sweetener (packet)	97	32

Reprinted with permission from The Calorie Control Council

SECTION 4

QUICK, EASY FOOD PLANNING AND PREPARATION

Did you ever give the excuse that you don't have time for meal planning and preparation on the way through the fast food line? Below are some tips that can save you time, improve your nutrition, and take time out of your busy schedule. Plan menus weekly to save time when shopping. Look at items you have on hand to avoid extra trips to the grocery. Then, check the foods you have on hand and use your shopping list to organize the foods you need. This will help you stick to your nutrition plan because planning ahead will reduce impulse ordering. When you've completed your meal plans for four separate weeks you'll notice quite a variety of foods. Planning a month of meal plans will allow variety and give you the ability to use them over and over again. At times, you may want to add new items that can be substituted for your favorites to prevent boredom with your meals and reflect seasonal variation.

MEAL PLANNING GUIDE: IT'S ALL ABOUT THE CHOICE

1. Keep a running list of the items that you need so that you are prepared when you start writing out your grocery list. This also saves extra trips to the grocery store.

2. Make sure that you plan your meals weekly and make a shopping list before you hit the grocery store. Planning will help you resist impulse buying that will save you money and improve your health.

3. Check out websites that provide menu planners, shopping lists, and recipes to make your planning easier.

4. Arrange your shopping list by category and then arrange the categories according to the layout of your supermarket. Many grocery chains do this already so check their websites or use the Weekly Meal Planning Guide in this chapter.

5. Know the layout of your grocery store so you can move up and down the aisles quickly.

6. Pick the correct number of servings from the five major food groups when planning your daily menus. Use www.Choose-MyPlate.gov, www.mealsmatter.org, and www.foodonthetable.com to guide your food selection.

7. Using a menu helps you to plan on using leftovers more effectively. They can be used for soups, sandwiches, or

casseroles during the week. Some of these items could be made on Sundays or put together quickly during the week. This is particularly useful for late nights at work when fatigue leads to impulse eating.

8. Select an entrée for each lunch and dinner. Use foods on hand to complement each meal.

Regardless of your shopping style, use the Weekly Menu Planning Guide first to save time and to make the best food decisions. Then, check the foods you have on hand and use your shopping list to organize the foods you need. Take into consideration if you will be eating at home or on the road. Fill in the out of town meals with ideas of what you will order.

BREAKFAST

	Sun	Mon	Tues	Weds	Thurs	Fri	Sat
Fruit or Juice Cereal or Starch							
Protein Bevarage and/or milk							

LUNCH

	Sun	Mon	Tues	Weds	Thurs	Fri	Sat
Entrée Vegetable							
Starch Fruit Bevarage and/or milk							

DINNER

	Sun	Mon	Tues	Weds	Thurs	Fri	Sat
Entrée							
Vegetable							
Starch							
Fruit							
Bevarage and/or milk							
Salad							
Dessert							

25 TIME-SAVINGS MEAL TIPS TO HELP WHEN MEAL PLANNING

1. Box soups are good to keep on hand. Add a grill cheese sandwich to soups without protein or add pieces of leftover turkey, chicken, ground beef, or chopped up beef for your protein needs. Remember to watch sodium content.

2. Salsa is great to add to meatloaf, omelets, and fish. When making meatloaf, make two and freeze one for future use.

3. Shredded 2% cheese can be added to eggs, tuna melts, and pasta.

4. Eggs are a perfect protein for a quick breakfast, lunch, or dinner.

5. Low fat Greek yogurt is a great choice for a breakfast or lunch protein. Most brands equal 2 ounces of protein. Add a starch and fruit choice to make a meal.

6. Low fat Greek yogurt is also an easy way to make fruit smoothies or can be added to ice cube trays for a frozen yogurt treat.

7. Yogurt is also a great addition to dry cereals like bran or granola.

8. Frozen berries kept on hand can be added to fruit smoothies for a quick breakfast.

9. Spice blends like McCormick already made up or making your own from online recipes adds spice to your meals.

10. Steel cut and rolled oats can be added to smoothies, home-made cookies, muffins, or cereal bars.

11. Always have a jar or two of tomato sauce. These are high in cancer-fighting lycopene. Check for those with lower sugar content. Add to chicken, shrimp, or cooked vegetables.

12. Canned tuna is always a good protein to add to bread, cold or hot pasta, or salads.

13. Frozen veggie mixes should always be kept on hand. In addition to reducing wastage, they can be added to stir-fry, pot pies, or as a complement to a meal.

14. Peanut, almond, sunflower, and tahini butters can be added to sandwiches, vegetables, fruit, and crackers.

15. Canned beans can be added to salads, salsas, soups, or stuff them into pitas or tortillas.

16. Pasta is a quick food choice to make a meal. Try those made with protein and fiber. Try angel hair pasta for the fastest preparation.

17. Whole chickens are a reasonable meat choice that is quick and easy to prepare. Throw into a crock pot or instant pot with low sodium broth. Add potatoes, green beans, and carrots during the last 20 minutes. Add a salad on the side and you have a complete meal.

18. Try some of the new pre-cooked starches that only need to be warmed up in the microwave. These include a variety of rice dishes, lentils, pasta, or quinoa. These can be bought off the grocery shelf or purchase on Amazon.

19. Frozen spinach is great to add to lasagna, manicotti, omelets, soups, salads, and as a side dish.

20. Manicotti, pasta and meat sauce, and lasagna are great choices for left-overs. They can be served later in the week or frozen for later use.

21. Cooked beef strips, chicken slices, and ground beef provide families with a quick and easy way to make stir-fry, tacos, pot pies, and casseroles.

22. Frozen fish is a good choice because fish is generally frozen and then thawed before selling. Fish is also quick to cook and to put on the table after a long day.

23. Always keep frozen ravioli on hand. Boil and pour on spaghetti sauce. Add a fresh salad.

24. Have a variety of frozen vegetables in the freezer to provide your necessary vitamins, minerals, and fiber when you are low on fresh choices. They are peeled, trimmed, and ready to cook.

25. Although pre-cut and washed vegetables and fruits are more expensive, they are worth the money if they eliminate the need to eat out or stop at a fast food restaurant. Buy pre-cut and washed stir-fry vegetables, salads, spinach, baby carrots, and pre-cut pineapple to save some time.

SHOPPING IT'S

"Don't eat anything your great-great grandmother wouldn't recognize as food. There are a great many food-like items in the supermarket your ancestors wouldn't even recognize as foods. Stay away from these."

— Michael Pollan

Grocery shopping trends have changed in the last 25 years. Surveys show that between 30-60% of men are doing the primary shopping, up from 14% in 1985. Whether this is due to more men having flexible work schedules or more couples sharing household duties, men's contribution to shopping has had a major impact. Some characteristics of the male shopper include:

- Tend to walk through all of the aisles exploring different food options.
- Spend more time shopping and are less hurried.
- Apt to impulse buy.
- Enjoy customizing and adding a personal touch.
- Appear to be more experimental and adventurous in their food purchasing.
- Shop around the store for the best price more than women.

- Ask for help less often and generally make a second sweep through the store.
- Less likely to shop for groceries online.

As many as 89% of Americans say their grocery shopping routine has changed since Covid 19. Less eating out and more cooking at home has driven this change. More families are planning, cooking and eating meals together. We think this is a great change.

But the shopping experience is different. There is less wandering up and down the aisles fueled by an urgency to get in and out of stores quickly.

Regardless of your shopping style or whether we are experiencing a pandemic or not, use the Weekly Menu Planning Guide first to save time and make the best food decisions. Then, check the foods you have on hand and use your shopping list to organize the foods you need. Take into consideration if you will be eating at home or on the road. Fill in the out of town meals with ideas of what you will order. To allow safety when shopping don't zig-zag or backtrack through the store. Bag your groceries yourself.

13 EASY SHOPPING TIPS FOR QUICK MEALS

1. Use seasonal fresh fruits and vegetables to keep your costs down.

2. Eat before shopping to reduce impulse buying caused by hunger.

3. Leave the kids home, if possible, to avoid food fights in the store and excessive demands that cost you more money.

4. If you can't leave the kids at home, beware of pressures to buy candy, cookies, or other treats in order to appease a complaining child. Bring lower calorie choices to the store with you that they can snack on. These would include: fresh fruit, graham crackers, pretzels, or popcorn.

5. Know the layout of your grocery store so you can move up and down the aisles quickly.

6. Avoid peak grocery shopping times particularly on the way home from work. Grocery shopping is heaviest between 5 and 7 PM. The slowest times are weekdays before 9AM and after 8PM to miss the crowds.

7. Cross off items as you select them. Sticking to your lists will reduce impulse buying.

8. Check labels to insure the purchase of the best buy. Ingredients must be listed in the order that they predominate. Example: A label listing water, gravy, potatoes, carrots, and beef contains the most water and the least amount of beef.

9. Pass items at the checkout and at waist level since they are designed for impulse buying.

10. Purchase packages based upon how quickly you're able to use them. Usually a larger package is more economical, unless it can't be used or stored before it spoils.

11. If you have problems limiting portion sizes, buy individual serving snack packs. When you are done with the package it is a reminder that you have eaten your allotted amount.

12. Shop for packaged goods and staples first. Shop for perishable foods and frozen food last. As you unpack your order put away perishables first. Always move older supplies forward and put new supplies in the back of your storage area.

13. Shop on days when foods are freshest and most plentiful, usually toward the end of the week.

NEW GROCERY SHOPPING TRENDS

In 2018, 18 million U.S. consumers choose a grocery app 49.6% up from 2017. It is predicted that grocery apps will rise to 30 million by 2022. Since the Covid 19 pandemic, the use of grocery apps has increased from 3-4% of grocery spending to 5-10%. Stores are now offering apps that interact between consumer phones and available shelf tags. Kroger has started a healthy app called Opt Up that tracks nutritional quality of food choices and recommends healthier options. This trend has been put on the back burner with Covid-19 as shoppers are shopping more quickly to reduce contact with others.

More grocery chains will offer restaurants for fast healthy eating. Grocery stores will increase the offering of private store labels in place of off brands. It is expected that in 5 years, store brand labels will show a 20-25% share of the market in contrast to off brand labels. This is expected because more shoppers will look for quality in products with a trust in their local grocery store.

Kroger has begun testing driverless deliveries in Arizona to reduce the cost and increase convenience to consumers. There have been a few mishaps that have slowed the expansion of this practice, but many areas are still using the drive-less deliveries.

Delivery services have not been popular with grocery shoppers. The biggest concern was the quality of produce. However; densely populated areas in the Northeast, West Coast, and the Pacific Northwest Washington State are more open to delivery services. These are being done mostly by Amazon that has a headquarters in Seattle.

In the South, most of the deliveries are being done by Wal-Mart or regional grocery stores. Wal-Mart presently has 1000 locations where deliveries are available. The Covid 19 pandemic has changed this a great deal as many people have reduced their grocery shopping with using delivery services. It has been anticipated that the use of delivery services will expand as more customers become accustomed and positive towards this time-saver.

FARMER'S MARKETS

Markets and community gardens are popping up all over, and we couldn't be more pleased. The trend to buy locally grown produce and foods is one many embrace but is certainly not new. Eleanor Roosevelt initiated the Community Gardens known as the *Victory Gardens of World War II*. Over 20 million gardens were planted and could be found on rooftops, in local parks, and private residences. Much like today, these markets supplied fresh foods, boosted moral, and connected people to each other and the land. In 2009, First Lady Michelle Obama encouraged healthy eating and natural foods with an initiative that included planting fruits and vegetables on the While House Lawn. Now, decades later, both city and rural areas offer Community Gardens. All that is required is a plot of land and a group of individuals with an interest in fresh, homegrown foods.

Farmers markets, on the other hand, are found at only certain locations within a community. They are often in cities and offer a variety of fresh produce, foods, and flowers brought in by local farmers.

According to the U. S. Department of Agriculture (USDA), in 2009, there were 5,274 farmers markets in the U.S., a 42% increase from the previous 5 years and an 84% increase since 2000. Some are seasonal, some year-around. For those of us who enjoy experiencing new foods and tasting, smelling, and touching our foods, farmers markets are a joy.

ACCORDING TO THE USDA, THESE ARE SOME ADVANTAGES TO SHOPPING AT FARMERS MARKETS:

- Enables growers and producers to develop personal relationships with customers
- Improves access to locally grown fresh produce
- Increases produce variety

9 TIPS TO GET THE MOST OUT OF FARMERS MARKETS:

- Make sure all vendors are growers/producers
- Shop early in the day for the best choices
- Shop seasonally
- Be prepared to spend more money for the value of some items
- Discover items not found at the local grocery store
- Ask how the foods were grown and processed
- Find out when the food was harvested
- Carry cash and a reusable shopping bags
- Get to know the seller/farmer (www.FruitandVeggieGuru.com)

COMMUNITY SUPPORTED AGRICULTURE

Community Supported Agriculture is not a new concept. In fact, it has been around for over 25 years. Farmers offer the opportunity to purchase fresh produce by buying "shares" from them. Seasonal produce including vegetables, fruits and sometimes honey, eggs dairy products and even flowers are available weekly from farmers throughout the season.

The American Journal of Public Health (June 2011) reported: More than half of those individuals who participated in community gardens met the nutrition recommendations to eat fruit and vegetables at least 5 times a day, compared to 37 percent of home gardeners and 25 percent of non-gardeners. The British Journal of Sports Medicine reports that daily gardening can reduce the risk of heart attack or stroke by 27% in adults over 60 years.

UNIQUE ADVANTAGES:

- Fresh food with all the flavor, vitamins and minerals
- Exposure to new vegetables and a new way of cooking
- May get to visit the farmer at least once a season
- Develop a relationship with the farmer who grows the foods.

For more information visit: www.localharvest.org/csa

Find a location near your home and enjoy the fresh, unprocessed foods of the lands which you will be pleased to know are not too far away (see websites below).

- www.localharvest.com
- www.ams.usda.gov/farmersmarkets
- www.epicurious.com
- www.pickyourown.org

SECTION 5

MEAL MANAGEMENT

BREAKFAST

Starting the day with breakfast is smart. Breakfast is good for you and there are many good reasons to slow down and take the time to eat breakfast. Research has shown that breakfast is the most important meal of the day and when consumed, people generally make better food choices later in the day. Those who eat breakfast also tend to get more fiber, calcium, riboflavin, zinc, iron, and vitamins A and C, as well as less fat and cholesterol. The American Journal of Clinical Nutrition reported in 2010 that those that skipped breakfast throughout childhood and as adults had higher levels of LDL (bad cholesterol) than those who had always eaten breakfast. The good news is that there are many fast, easy, and nutritious foods available that make starting the day with breakfast a no-brainer.

REVVING YOUR ENGINE

Breakfast means literally "break the fast." When we wake up after a night's sleep, we are in a fasting state (or starvation mode). You can jump start your metabolism by eating something first thing in the morning. When we eat something we literally wake up the digestive system, stimulating our metabolism. Skipping breakfast causes individuals to remain in a fasting state resulting in slower metabolism and the potential to interfere with weight loss efforts.

Many people complain to us that they just aren't hungry in the morning. More often than not, they've eaten a late dinner or snacked at bedtime. By avoiding eating late at night you'll be more likely to wake up hungry and look forward to breakfast. If you just don't care to eat first thing in the morning, plan to have something one or two hours after you get up. If you are stopping at your favorite fast food restaurant, know that there are healthy breakfast choices such as an egg white English muffin sandwich, fruit smoothies, and low-fat yogurts with fresh fruit. Or alternatively, bring a light morning snack to work like a piece of fruit, low- fat cheese, crackers, or a low-fat yogurt with low-fat granola or nuts.

After years of working with overweight patients, we have found that individuals who skip breakfast tend to overeat later in the day. They also tend to select foods higher in sugar and fat. When people select high-fiber breakfast foods, they typically find themselves feeling less hungry during the day and later evening. As a result, there is an overall lower caloric consumption and a spreading out of calories throughout the day which has been shown to be healthier for the body and soul.

New research done in 2013 has shown that skipping breakfast can lead to a 27 percent increase in the risk of heart disease. The research was conducted in 27,000 health care workers.

Skipping breakfast was found to increase the consumption of lost calories not consumed at breakfast to unhealthy eating during the rest of the day. It was also surmised that some individuals may place their bodies in a state of stress that affects metabolism and cardiovascular health.

Research conducted at the Monash University in Melbourne showed that it is likely to make no difference whether we skip breakfast or consume it. Researchers found that those who skip breakfast showed significant weight loss versus those who didn't. They found that individuals who consumed breakfast ate more calories during the day.

Research has also found that eating breakfast can improve school and work performance. Eating breakfast can aid with the following:

- Help with problem-solving, alertness, memory, and learning
- Increase scores on creativity tests
- Allow attentiveness, retention of material, and increased interest in learning new things
- Improve mood, increase calmness, and reduce stress

Interestingly, an increased carbohydrate intake is associated with improved mood. The B vitamins, folate, and thiamin, have also been found to improve mood, and thiamin has been found to increase feelings of well-being. For all of these reasons, it is important to incorporate eating breakfast into your busy day.

BREAKFAST TIPS

Breakfast can be easily packed with nutrition by discovering a few healthy items that are easy to prepare and that you enjoy. It is also one of the quickest and easiest meals to put together since many breakfast foods do not require cooking. Make sure you include protein in your meal. Aim for at least 5 grams of protein for a balance of nutrients and to prevent those feelings of hunger that can appear two to three hours after an all carbohydrate meal. A breakfast with some protein and high-quality carbohydrates that have fiber can aid in weight loss efforts by keeping you feeling fuller longer.

Scramble some egg whites or egg beaters and sandwich them between some whole grain toast or English muffin. Don't forget that an 8 oz. glass of orange juice fortified with calcium and vitamin D will provide 120% of your vitamin C, 35% of your calcium, and 25% of your vitamin D daily requirements.

You can drink your breakfast by making a fruit smoothie, combining low fat milk or yogurt and fresh fruit, or drinking an already prepared beverage. You can add protein powder to a beverage for added protein. Check the beverage section for more information on smoothies. Here are some suggestions for easy nutritious breakfasts:

- Top breakfast cereals with fresh, frozen, canned, or dried fruits: pineapple, bananas, berries, raisins, cranberries, dates, or apricots.
- Mix a variety of breakfast cereals together to give a mixture of tastes and textures. Look for high fiber breakfast cereals. At least 5 grams.
- Add nuts to cereal (hot or cold for a crunchy texture).
- For a taste of sweetness, try a teaspoon of chocolate chips or five mini- marshmallows.
- Add low-fat granola or nuts to your low-fat yogurt.
- Hard boiled eggs
- Peanut butter on an apple (refrigerate for a few minutes)
- Many people forget that vegetables can also be added to breakfast. Drink a glass of tomato juice or load your omelet with tomatoes, broccoli, spinach, or asparagus. Or cut up raw vegetables to add to your meal.

Try some non-traditional types of food for breakfast such as the following:

- Grilled cheese (and tomato) sandwich, peanut butter and banana sandwich, peanut butter on raisin toast or whole grain bread, cottage cheese or plain yogurt with fresh or canned fruit, hard cooked eggs, or mozzarella sticks.
- Breakfast pizza or use leftover pizza.
- Try some typical dessert items such as rice pudding with a reduced amount of sugar.

- Low-fat cheese chunks with fresh fruit such as grapes or apple slices.
- Make your own breakfast cereal bars.
- Whole wheat English muffins with low-fat cheese, peanut butter, or Canadian bacon
- Glucerna Bars or Shakes
- Carnation Instant Breakfast
- Slim-Fast Shakes
- Nutrition bars (see the Digging the Bar Facts chapter)

CHOOSING BREAKFAST CEREALS

It is important to watch the sugar content of cereals selected. Manufacturers of breakfast cereals pay a lot of money to obtain grocery store shelf space that will enhance your choice of particular types of cereals. Sugary cereals are generally at shopping cart level where children will see them and attempt to convince their parents to purchase the cereals advertised during the Saturday morning cartoon's commercials. At the adult eye level, we find sweetened adult cereals that tempt us to make impulsive decisions. In general, the top shelf contains the healthier choices, along with those that boast of being healthier (but in reality, are not).

To help you make the right decision for healthy cereals, focus on these key label items:

- serving size
- fiber
- calories
- carbohydrate and sugar content

The weight of a serving is generally 30 grams, but can vary from one-third to two cups depending on the cereal's fluffiness and packaging of the flakes. A good portion size for the average person is one and a half cups of cereal. Athletes will generally consume at least three cups of cereal at one time.

High fiber cereals are those that provide four grams of fiber per serving and very high fiber cereals contain six grams of fiber or more. Remember that you should consume 25- 40 grams of fiber each day.

A cereal's sugar content is very important when selecting a breakfast cereal. Check the label for the *total carbohydrate* content. Under this heading look for sugar. This is how much sugar (in grams) that is in one serving of your cereal. Every 4 grams of sugar on the label is the equivalent to adding a teaspoon of sugar to the cereal. If a cereal label states it contains 14 grams of sugar that is the equivalent of 3 ½ teaspoons of sugar.

Dietitians and dentists recommend that you choose cereals that contain fewer than 6 grams of sugar per serving. Childhood obesity and tooth decay are two health risks that can be decreased with reduction of sugar intake. There are more than 40 breakfast cereals on the market that contain 6 grams of sugar or less. Government guidelines recommend that any cereal with sugar content greater than 10% of calories in a serving is too high in sugar. For example, if a cereal contains 160 calories, it should not contain more than 16 calories or one teaspoon of sugar.

You can piece together a healthy, well-balanced breakfast that takes just a few minutes. Try and include at least two or three of the following: whole grains, low-fat dairy, low-fat protein and fruits or vegetables when possible. We hope breakfast becomes a natural part of your day.

LUNCH AND DINNER BAGS

When you are too busy to go out for lunch or dinner, bag lunches and dinners can be a smart idea. The advantage of bag meals is that you are controlling what you're eating and not worrying about what is added to the food. If you can bring a bag lunch or dinner to work, on the way to an appointment, or when running errands, your calories will be more easily managed. A bagged meal will be especially helpful if you are on the road and unfamiliar with local restaurants.

Bag lunches and dinners can get boring if the same sandwich is packed each day. Try adding variety by varying the type of sandwich fillings, breads, spreads, and sauces. If you have access to a microwave and refrigerator, a frozen lunch or dinner is a good option. Try adding a fruit, vegetable, and possibly a starch serving to frozen meals.

Varied Sandwich Ideas	
Eggs	Medium to Hard Poached, Scrambled, Hard-cooked
Fillers	Lettuce - try varying the type, Tomato, Red Onion, Avocado Slices, Sauerkraut, Chopped Apple, Chopped Nuts, Olives, Bacon Bits
Spreads	Regular and Lite Mayonnaise, Flavored Mayonnaise (e.g. chipotle), Dijonnaise, Barbeque Sauce, Mustard, Honey Mustard, Catsup, Chili Sauce, Sour Cream (Lite or Regular), Horseradish Sauce
Reduced Fat Cheeses	Cheddar, Colby, Mozzarella Sticks Cream Cheese, Swiss, Processed Cheese,
Sandwich Salads (Low-Fat Mayonnaise)	Chicken, Corned Beef, Crabmeat, Egg, Salmon, Shrimp, Tuna (water-packed), Turkey

EASY MEALS: THE QUICK OF IT

Quick Meal Preparation

Slow-Cooker / Instant Pot / Multicooker

The slow cooker remains a helpful appliance for our fast-paced lives. It can be started before leaving for work, and dinner – or a good portion of it -- is ready when we get home. The slow cooker is ideal for tougher, cheaper cuts of meat and is easy to clean.

The Instant Pot and other multicookers are a new take on the slow cooker. They have the functions of a pressure cooker, rice cooker, steamer, yogurt-maker, and hard-egg cooker. They can also sterilize baby bottles.

Which One is Best

Consumer Reports found that the slow cooker and Instant Pot performed similarly in tests. The slow cooker is usually much cheaper and easier to clean. The Instant Pot produces a thicker yogurt. Either is a great choice to help busy families produce quick and easy meals.

Mason Jar Meals

Using mason jars to prep meals can save time and produce healthier and more attractive meals. For salads, layer protein such as chicken, tuna, beans, and nuts with lettuce and a variety of other vegetables. It allows you to create multiple meals ahead of time for lunches and dinners. Mason jars are cheap, readily available, and easy to clean. Some people eat their meal right out of the jar while others use a plate to dish out their meal from the jar. Mason jars are also useful for breakfast. Cook hot cereal the night before or on the weekend and layer cereal, nuts, and fruits in the jar. This makes it easy in the morning to spoon out the meal and then race out the door or take the jar with you to eat breakfast at work.

Sheet Pan Dinners

The entire meal is made on a sheet pan or cookie sheet. Line the pan with foil or parchment paper for easy clean up. Season and place protein on one section of the pan. Chop vegetables into uniform pieces, coat with oil and seasonings and place on sheet pan with protein. Roast in the oven until cooked through. For vegetables that require less time in the oven, add them part way through the cooking process.

Air Fryers

Air fryers are another way to cook fast, healthy foods. They are similar to ovens because they bake and roast. The difference is that there is a large, powerful fan on top that allows food to become super crispy in little time. They heat very quickly and use little or no oil. Most air fryers are easy to clean either in your dishwasher or with a brush.

Recipes are online with many great ideas to mix and match to your personal tastes.

Frozen Meals

When you go down the frozen food aisle, you will notice that frozen meals are the most popular items. To insure you make the best choices, check the nutrition label. The brands that tend to be the healthiest are: Healthy Choice, Smart Ones, and Lean Cuisine. These meals tend to be lower in sodium, fat, and calories.

When you are picking a brand, make sure that the meal you pick gives nutrition information based on the whole package. Check for a good amount of vegetables, higher fiber grains like brown rice, wild rice, couscous, or quinoa. Other healthy starch choices include beans, peas, corn, and whole wheat pasta.

Tips for Picking a Frozen Meal:

1. Pick a meal that contains less than 800 mg. sodium each that is a third of the 2300 mg daily sodium you should be striving for.

2. Keep meals to less than 250-300 calories each. An extra starch may be needed if carbohydrate is less than 30 grams for the meal.

3. Choose meals with less than 4 grams of saturated fat.

4. Select meals with 3-5 grams fiber and make sure to add a salad and fresh fruit that will get your fiber intake to one third of your daily need.

* 25 grams fiber for women and 35 grams for men

Even better than selecting a frozen meal is making your own. Although busy people do not think they can fit this into their hectic schedules, planning ahead can make this a no brainer!

The most important thing to consider is that making your own frozen meals will allow you complete control over what is in the meal. It will allow you to restrict salt, artificial ingredients, preservatives, and unhealthy fats often present in the best-frozen meals. You can make your meals with brown rice in place of white rice, use more vegetables, and cook with healthier olive oil. The cost of frozen meals starts to add up and adds approximately $100 to your monthly budget.

Making your own frozen meals does not have to be time-consuming. Some people will put aside a day a month to make meals. Others, like us, use leftovers from meals cooked to provide frozen dinners for later use during the week. It is often easier to cook an extra serving when cooking a meal to be used at a later meal.

Another advantage of making your own meals is that they are more ecofriendly. Frozen dinners are packed in plastic and cardboard that winds up in landfills. By making your own at home, you can decrease your impact on the planet by using glass or plastic containers that can be used more than once.

Making your own meals insures variety because you are controlling what is put in the meal. This allows you to pick favorite entrees and vegetables that you might not like in a frozen meal. This allows you to change the menu, ingredients, and the meal combinations and also provides you a chance to try new recipes.

When making your own meals, the containers you use should be microwave and freezer-safe. Check the website: www.nrdc.org to insure container safety. You can find a variety of safe divided containers from Amazon, Wal-Mart and the Container Store.

Before you portion out the food, allow prepared food to cool completely and leave room at the top of the container to allow expansion of food during freezing. Insure that the food is wrapped and covered with airtight lids to prevent air from getting in. Items that have high moisture content, like soups freeze better than drier foods.

Mark the food with a permanent marker with the item name and date made. Use each meal within a couple of weeks to insure maximum quality and flavor.

Vegetables should be slightly undercooked to prevent mushiness when reheated.

Make sure that hot food is cooled before freezing to prevent the growth of bacteria.

Use your frozen meals within 3 months to insure safety and freshness. And trust your instincts. If it does not smell right or tastes "off", THROW OUT! Defrosted food should not be refrozen because you will risk bacterial contamination.

Meal Kits

Meal kits are a new way for those too busy to prepare meals to eat fast and healthy. It has been estimated that 20% of Americans have tried meal kits in this last year.

They provide the ingredients necessary to prepare a meal that is time-saving and can save you money. This eliminates having unused items that you might never use again.

Meal kits are helpful for families because putting a meal together displays deep emotional needs that are at play. Instead of pulling items out of bags, the family, couple, or single has a deeper connection to the food. They also begin to experiment with cooking that may be their first time preparing a meal. A greater satisfaction is derived from this type of meal preparation that is not derived from take-out food.

There are a number of meal kit companies available. Blue Apron is the largest company and is the most well-known. They attempted to sell their meal kits at Costco, but had to discontinue the program due to financial loss. They are still offering the meals online for delivery to homes. Amazon offers meal kits for online order and delivery as well as meal kits to buy at Whole Foods. Sun Basket is another meal kit that is similar to Amazon, but the foods are all organic.

It is important to realize that you need to check with your regular grocery to see what if any meal kits are available. It will be interesting to see how meal kits fare. It is a helpful addition for families who want to eat healthy but don't have the time to do it. But the future of meal kits will be dependent on price, possible boredom with foods provided, and the training of individuals to learn how to cook quick and easy meals.

Easy Dinner Meal Recipes

Coming home from work or a busy afternoon carpooling should not eliminate the possibility of putting a home cooked meal on the table. Planning out your menus in advance makes it possible to do some of the work ahead of time. This will enable you to cut down meal preparation when you hit the door.

Time how long it takes you to make a stop at a take-out or fast food restaurant. Then time how long it takes you to put something easy together. Browning meat can be done the night before when you are washing dishes or in the morning when making lunches. When you have food available for leftovers, cut up the meat and decide how you will use it for another meal.

The following are just a few ideas for quick and easy meals:

Spaghetti with lean beef/ turkey/marinara sauce	Put ground beef or ground turkey in a micro- wave safe baking dish. Break up into small pieces. Microwave until brown. Take out and drain off fat. Add water and drain. Pat dry. Add tomato sauce and microwave until warm.
Lean hamburg- ers or turkey burgers on a bun	Throw lean hamburgers in a frying pan or grill and brown.
Grilled tuna sandwich on a bun or English muffin	Mix one 5-ounce can of tuna with lite mayo. Top with a slice of 2% fat cheese. (makes two servings)
Cooked beef, chicken, pork, fish, or bean fajitas	Cook peppers and onions in a skillet with olive oil or cooking sprays. Add to cooked meal entrée choice. Add 2% fat grated cheese and place on a tortilla.
Cooked chicken, beef, fish or bean tacos	Add cooked protein entrée choice to a soft or hard tortilla. Add grated 2% cheese.
Kraft Macaroni and Cheese Cas- serole (mostly for the kids!)	Add lean cooked ground meat or turkey meat, ham chunks, chicken, or tuna. Add cooked frozen vegetables. Follow directions on pack- age, use lite margarine and skim milk to reduce calories. Combine ingredients in a casserole. Sprinkle the top with breadcrumbs. Bake in the oven for 20 minutes to combine flavors.

Barbequed pork on a light hamburger bun	If you have cooked a lean pork loin on the grill and have leftovers: Add barbeque sauce and a little water and cook until warm. Place on a lite hamburger bun.
Grilled Vegetables	Wash zucchini, eggplant, and/or carrots. Slice them large enough, through the width, so that they won't fall through the grill rack. Brush or drizzle with olive oil. Let each slice brown then remove them from the rack. Cut to desired serving size, or dice and add them to couscous or brown rice.
Cottage cheese and fruit and a large roll	Put ½ c. low-fat cottage cheese and fruit in a bowl. Add a large roll on the side.
Grilled beef, chicken, turkey, ham, pork, or lamb	Add any of these meats to grill. Cook until meat is cooked to preferred doneness. Add some grilled vegetables and a starch choice for a complete meal.
Grilled cheese sandwich (2% fat cheese) and cup of soup	Add low-fat margarine to two slices of bread. Add cheese and place in frying pan. Brown on one side and then the other. Open up a can of soup and warm or add a homemade soup made in advance.
Hot turkey/beef sandwich with low fat gravy	Warm up turkey or beef leftovers or buy turkey or beef at the deli counter. Warm with low-fat gravy. Place turkey or beef on sandwich bread with hot gravy.
Chili	Add 8 ounces of tomato sauce and a 26-ounce can of stewed tomatoes to the browned meat. Add 4 cans of kidney beans drained, a large cut up green pepper, a medium cut up onion, and 3 tbs. of chili powder. Cook in a slow cooker or instant pot on either high or low depending on your needs.

Chili macaroni	Add ½ cup of cooked macaroni to a ½ cup of warmed chili.
Chicken, ham, tuna salad, roast beef or turkey roll-up	Place protein entrée choice on tortilla. See Roll-ups/Wraps for further suggestions.
Bean, rice, and 2% cheese roll-up	Drain beans from can and warm in the microwave oven. Cook rice until done. Add grated 2% fat cheese. Roll ingredients in a tortilla. Try higher fiber tortillas for reduced calories.
Stuffed baked potato with 2% cheese and broccoli	Wash a potato. Poke with holes. Put a wet paper towel around the potato and place in microwave at microwave timing. Cook broccoli in microwave until cooked. Place 2% cheese on top of cooked baked potato and cook for 45 seconds. Top with hot broccoli.

Pasta Meals

LOW FAT WHITE SAUCE

188 calories, 8 gr. of carbohydrates,12.1 gr. of protein, 12 gr. of fat

Ingredients:

- 1tbs. healthy margarine choice
- 2 tsp. all-purpose flour
- 2 small cloves garlic, minced
- 1 1/3 cups skim milk
- 2 tbs. lite cream cheese
- 1 cup freshly grated Parmesan cheese/2 tsp. fresh parsley

Directions: Melt margarine in a saucepan over medium heat. Add garlic and sauté for 1 minute. Stir in the flour and gradually add milk stirring with a wire whisk until it is blended. Cook approximately 8 minutes until thickened and bubbly stirring constantly. Add lite cream cheese and cook for 2 minutes. Add 1 cup of Parmesan cheese, stirring constantly, until melted. Add parsley. Makes 4 servings.

PASTA DINNERS

Combine the items under the following categories to give you various pasta dinners.

- **Pasta/Starch**

  Whole wheat pasta any type(spaghetti, linguini, penne, ziti, etc)

  White pasta any type (spaghetti, linguini, penne, ziti, etc)

  Angel hair pasta cooks fast- approximately 3-5 minutes

- **Protein**

  Grilled Chicken Breast

  Ground Turkey/Beef Beef/ Pork chunks

  Grilled Salmon

  Shrimp/Scallops/Mussels/ Clams

  Turkey/Chicken sausage

  Smart Ground - soy meat substitute/Water-packed Tuna

- **Veggies**

  Tomatoes

  Zucchini

  Eggplant

  Edamame

  Mushrooms

  Sundried Tomatoes

  Cauliflower

  Broccoli

- **Sauces**

  Marinara

  White wine Pesto

  Italian dressing

  Garlic/butter

  White sauce

  Olive Oil

- **Add-Ins**
  Bread Crumbs

- **Spices**
  Cloves

  Cinnamon sticks

  Low-Fat grated Cheese

  Crushed red-pepper/Garlic powder

ROLL-UPS & WRAPS

Combine the items under the following categories to give you various wraps.

- **Protein**

  Chicken

  Lean Beef

  Salmon

  Tuna

  Water-packed Tuna

  Pork

  Beans

  Grated Cheese - can be used alone or as a topping for the other proteins

- **Wraps & Tortillas**

  Spinach

  Flour

  Wheat

  Black Bean

- **Fillers**

  Lettuce

  Spinach

  Sugar snap peas

  Fresh Cilantro

  Carrots

  Cabbage

  Raisins

  Cranberries

  Mushrooms

  Black Olives

  Tomato

- **Spreads**

Light Mayo	Honey Dijon
Spicy Brown Mustard	Avocado
Yellow Mustard	Salsa
Light Cream Cheese	Light Italian Dressing
Low-Fat grated Cheese	Other Light Salad Dressings
Crushed red-pepper	Hummus
	Garlic powder

STIR-FRY MEALS

STIR-FRY RECIPES GETTING STARTED:

1. Heat your wok or skillet over low heat.
2. Marinate your protein choice in 1 tbsp. light soy sauce and 1 tbsp. dry or sweet sherry. This can be done while cutting the produce chosen.
3. Cut produce.
4. Mince 1 tbsp. of garlic and ginger root.
5. Mix 2 tsp. cornstarch and 2 tbs. chicken broth or water.
6. Spray skillet or wok with Cooking Spray.
7. Stir-fry your protein choice until brown.
8. Add minced garlic and ginger root.
9. Add protein to wok or skillet.
10. Coat with any of the below sauces.
11. Stir in cornstarch mixture until juices are saucy and glossy. If the sauce appears too thick, add more chicken broth or water.
12. Serve the protein, produce, and sauce with rice, noodles, pasta, or couscous.

FRESH CILANTRO STIR-FRY SAUCE

- **Ingredients:**

  ¼ cup chicken broth

  ¼ cup light soy sauce / 2 tsp. rice wine vinegar

  ½ tsp. sugar or 1 tsp. artificial sweetener

  ¼ cup minced cilantro leaves

- **Directions:** Mix together ingredients in a 1-cup measuring cup and pour over stir-fry mixture stirring frequently. Calories are negligible for each serving. Makes 4 servings.

SWEET & SOUR STIR-FRY SAUCE

- **Ingredients:**

  ¼ cup chicken broth   2 tbs. light soy sauce

  2 tbs. rice wine vinegar   1 tbs. brown sugar

  ½ tsp. hot red pepper flakes

- **Directions:** Mix ingredients together in a 1-cup measuring cup and pour over stir-fry mixture stirring frequently. Contains approximately 12 calories and 3 grams of carbohydrate for each serving. Makes 4 servings.

LEMON STIR-FRY SAUCE

- **Ingredients:**

  ¼ cup chicken broth   1 tsp. lemon zest

  ¼ cup lemon juice   2 tbs. light soy sauce

  2 tbs. sugar or 2 tbs. sugar substitute

- **Directions:** Mix together ingredients together in a 1-cup measuring cup. Pour over stir-fry mixture stirring frequently. Contains approximately 25 calories and 6 grams carbohydrate per serving. Using a sugar substitute in place of sugar reduces calories to negligible. Makes 4 servings.

SESAME SOY SAUCE

- **Ingredients:**

  ¼ cup chicken broth   2 tsp. rice vinegar

  ¼ cup light soy sauce   1 tsp. sesame oil

  1 tsp. red pepper flakes   1 tsp. sugar

- **Directions:** Mix ingredients together in a 1-cup measuring cup. Pour over stir-fry mixture stirring frequently. Contains approximately 8 calories and 2 grams of carbohydrate per serving. Using a sugar substitute in place of sugar reduces the calories to negligible.

ᴳ HONEY SOY SAUCE

- **Ingredients:**

  ¼ cup honey   1 tbs. orange zest

  ½ cup rice vinegar   1 tsp. red pepper flakes

  2 tbs. light soy sauce

- **Directions:** Mix ingredients together in a 1-cup measuring cup. Pour over stir-fry mixture stirring frequently. Contains approximately 70 calories and 18 grams of carbohydrate per serving. Makes 4 servings.

STIR-FRY COMBOS

Stir-fry cooking can provide numerous quick meals. Mixing the groups below will provide many menu ideas.

- **Protein**

Chicken Strips	Shrimp Scallops
Pork Chunks	Beef Strips / Tofu

- **Starch**

Wild Rice	White Rice
Noodles	Couscous
Noodles	Pasta Quinoa

- **Flavorings**

La Choy Soy	Sesame Oil
Garlic / Ginger	Sauce

- **Nuts**

Peanuts / Cashews	Light Soy Sauce

- **Vegetables**

  Green, Red, and Yellow Peppers

Broccoli	Celery
Sugar snap peas	Scallions
Asparagus	Onions
Zucchini	Frozen Stir-Fry Vegetables
Mushrooms	

- **Directions:** Cook rice or rice noodles. Add vegetable spray to skillet and add protein choice until thoroughly cooked. Remove protein from skillet and move to the side. Add vegetables to skillet cooking until tender for about 3-4 minutes. Put protein back into the skillet with vegetables and add flavorings, heating for 1 extra minute.

DINING OUT

"The more you eat, the less the flavor;
the less you eat, the more the flavor."

— *Chinese Proverb*

Dining Out Questions: Test your knowledge of dining out by answering True or False to the questions below.

1. You cannot follow a healthy diet when you eat out.

2. Fast foods can never be eaten if you are trying to lose weight.

3. Layering a meal with a variety of foods will only cause you to eat too many calories.

4. The average American eats out one or two times per week.

5. Alcohol can fill you up and diminish your appetite.

Let's face it. Eating out frequently means we increase our chances of eating more calories and gaining weight. Serving sizes in many restaurants are bigger than ever. Dinner plates, like portion sizes, have grown. What ever happened to the 8-inch dinner plate? The average dinner plate is now around 12 inches and chefs are happy to pile on the portions.

A study in the Journal of Obesity, 2007, reported when chefs were interviewed, they stated, "regular size" portions are served 76% of the time. In reality, "regular size" portions of steak and pasta are 2 to 4 times larger than the serving size recommended by the U.S. Government. Planning your meals in advance and establishing reliable strategies can help you make good choices and eat healthy while dining out.

Learn to navigate restaurant menus. Most restaurants will accommodate requests to order from the children's menu, split a meal, or choose ala Carte. By ordering ala Carte you can easily piece together a meal that meets your nutrition goals. If it is difficult to piece together a reduced calorie meal then plan on taking a doggie bag home, or like some individuals, simply eat half.

If you eat out frequently, look at www.HealthyDiningFinder.com to identify menu items that fit into your eating plan.

A DAY AT A GLANCE

Take time out before you start the day to look at your schedule and the different eating situations you will be confronted with. If you are going to dine out, think about what you will be eating the rest of the day. When you plan your week of menus make sure you include low calorie items to balance the days and meals you may not be able to control. Try not to skip meals; the empty hunger will cause you to eat more. Instead, if you are eating out for dinner, eat a smaller lunch. Plan an afternoon snack to take the edge off your appetite.

FAST FOODS

Fast foods are just that: fast. The USDA's research study of 9,000 Americans shows that about a quarter of US adults over the age of 20 eat fast foods and drink twice as many sugary drinks than those who do not. That translates into more calories, fats, carbohydrates, proteins, and added sugars than those that do not. Adding 100 kcal per day can add 10 lbs. to your waistline in one year.

Choose smart. The good news is fast foods come in all shapes and sizes and are available just about everywhere. When you're on the road or in a hurry there's nothing wrong with stopping at a fast food restaurant. If you are going to be eating on the road carry a fast food calorie guide. Calorie King is a good choice, and can be purchased at most bookstores and on Amazon. (Check the References section of this book for some available guides.) Though fast foods are generally high in calories, fat, and sodium, by using the available nutrition information you can find healthy alternatives. Pay attention to the number of calories in a serving. The reason most fast foods are high in calories is because they are high in fat. Fat has 9 calories per gram, while carbohydrates and proteins have only 4 calories. So food choices that are high in fat tend to be high calorie items.

An advantage to eating at a fast food restaurant is nutrition information is often available to the consumer. Most fast food restaurants have low calorie healthy items. Subway's menu includes several sandwiches that average 300 calories, so even with a bag of baked chips and a diet soda a lunch can total less than 500 calories. Avoiding the super-size items saves calories. A plain hamburger, small fries, and diet coke can also fit into a meal plan. Salads and soups are also available. Piece a meal together by adding up the calories.

MANAGING A MENU

Put together a meal that is enjoyable, healthy, and fits into your calorie budget by using this planning checklist:

1. Try to avoid waiting for a table. Make a reservation and be on time. You can save yourself a few hundred calories by avoiding pre-dinner drinks and appetizers.

2. Think about how you want to "spend" your calories before beginning to scan the menu in a restaurant. You can also

research the restaurant's menu ahead of time in order to avoid making an impulsive decision.

3. Review all the menu items available, and work your way through from appetizers to desserts. Choose foods that are healthy and enjoyable. Don't let others pressure you into ordering foods you really don't need or want. Be polite and firm and stick to your plan.

4. Don't be shy about asking how food is prepared. Most restaurants are happy to share this information with you.

5. Modify menu items or substitute low calorie alternatives. Restaurants are used to requests to hold the sauce, go light on the dressing, or put the dressings and gravies on the side. These steps can save you calories.

6. Ask for baked items instead of fried. Most restaurants don't use the "good" fats anyway, so why take in extra fat, especially if it isn't the healthy kind. There are smart choices you can make about the kind of fat you use.

Remember to determine your hunger level and order your meal accordingly. An appetizer and side dish can be combined to make an entrée. If the appetizer is small, order two appetizers instead of an entire meal. Split your meal with a dining partner, plan to take some home for the next day, or simply leave it. You should be eating until you are satisfied. Listen to your body's signals and become attuned to when you are getting full. Eat slowly and enjoy the company of those you are with.

DRINKS

Regular sodas, lemonade, alcohol, or any beverage that is sweetened can easily add lots of calories. You're better off with a diet beverage or an unsweetened iced tea. You might want to avoid alcohol if it isn't that important to you. Besides, you may find that alcohol stimulates your appetite.

Since alcohol can make you less aware of what you are eating, you also run the risk of eating more than you had planned. If you do decide to drink, avoid mixed drinks (alcohol mixed with a caloric beverage, such as a soda or fruit juice). A better choice is a glass of red or white wine or hard liquor mixed with a non-caloric beverage such as club soda or diet soda. Ask the bartender to "go easy" on the hard liquor. You can save yourself 100 calories or more a drink.

Learn to limit your alcohol to one drink and sip that drink alternating with water throughout the meal. The calorie level of several drinks can add up quickly and can be equal to the calories of a small meal. Alcohol contains 7 calories per gram. So drinks containing alcohol tend to be high calorie items with little if any nutritional value.

APPETIZERS

Beware of appetizers. They are often high in fat and calories. Many appetizers are fried and breaded making them high calorie items. Sometimes it is best to avoid appetizers entirely. Consider splitting an appetizer with your dining partner. Low calorie items such as soups (broth-based), vegetables, and fruits are good options. Avoid creamy soups, sauces, and dips. Seafood, if it isn't fried, is a good choice. Combining a drink or two and a high calorie appetizer will add as many as 400 calories before you've even started your meal.

LAYER YOUR MEAL

Meal layering is helpful in making you feel fuller with less food. Try to start your meal with a lower calorie, high fiber food. Fresh vegetables, vegetable soup, or a salad with low calorie dressing will fit the bill. The American Journal of Clinical Nutrition reports that people who eat vegetables with a meal actually consume 20 percent fewer calories overall. Eat slowly enough to allow for the 20-minute interval where your body signals the brain that there is food in the stomach. If you eat large quantities of food before the 20-minute interval, you are not allowing enough time for your brain to receive the signal that there is food present in the stomach. This leads to overeating.

BREAD

Though the breadbasket seems to be the dieter's demise, who doesn't like a slice of warm crusty French or Italian bread with a meal? Actually a slice of bread contains only 60 to 80 calories and can easily be part of a meal plan. The problem is that limiting yourself to one or two slices often isn't easy. Remember also that adding butter, oil or Parmesan cheese can turn an innocent slice of bread into a high calorie item. Try eating a slice of bread without any topping and limiting it to one or two slices. If your will power takes a beating, ask the waitress to remove the breadbasket or move it away. Providing patrons with a breadbasket is a restaurant's way of keeping you busy while you wait for your meal. Fill the time with water, a low- calorie drink, or conversation. Don't get pressured into eating foods that you really don't want or need. Have a plan and stick to it.

SIDE DISHES

Side dishes are a compliment to an entree and should be modest in portion size. Salads can fool. We tend to think of them as low-calorie items, and indeed salads without a high calorie dressing can be a good filler before the meal begins. But a low-calorie salad can become 250 calories or more if you douse it liberally with dressing. Ask about substituting side dishes if the entrée you choose comes with high calorie choices. You can often trade in a double baked potato or fried potatoes for wild rice pilaf, or a plain baked potato, or skip it all together. Choose vegetables without sauces and avoid gravies. Most restaurants will be happy to make the switch for you. Fresh vegetables are low calorie, high in fiber, fill you up, and provide healthy nutrition.

ENTER THE ENTRÉE

The varieties of entrées to choose from are usually extensive providing an opportunity to eat healthy. Consider the portion size. Pastas are usually served in large quantities. Add a cream sauce and it becomes an even higher calorie item.

Ravioli and lasagna meals have fillings and sauces that may make them high in calories. Consider splitting an entrée with a friend or keep half for the next day's lunch. Pasta served with a grilled vegetable or with a fresh tomato sauce will save you lots of calories.

A grilled, 16 oz. steak may sound delicious, but it packs a mountain of calories into the one item. The steak alone can provide as many as 800 calories. Instead, try a small 4-6 oz. filet. This can save you as many as 400 calories. A half-roasted chicken might initially appeal to you as a possible dinner choice. You might think it's a menu item thought of as low calorie and healthy. Yet the reality is this portion is enough for two people, or lunch for two days. If you wouldn't eat half a chicken at home, try to limit the portion size when eating out. Fresh fish, especially if it's the "special of day" can be a great choice. If you don't like to cook fish at home, ordering it when you eat out provides a healthy and low-calorie alternative to many other menu items. Remember, fish contains the right kind of fat. However, be sure you know how it is prepared. Avoid fried fish, especially if coated in a batter. The added calories and fat of batter coated fried fish turns this healthy choice into a calorie nightmare. Grilled and baked fish will save lots of calories. Keep sauces on the side, and eat sparingly. Sauces and toppings are usually made from a fat source and hide the true flavor of foods especially fish. Ask for sauces on the side and use them sparingly.

Design your own meal. Break from tradition and order an appetizer, or a few appetizers to share with friends, to use as your entrée. Try an antipasti plate that comes with a variety of meats, cheese, and olives. A slice of bread, salad, and a glass of wine makes for a great dinner. Tapas are popular and you'll have a fun meal and leave the restaurant not feeling stuffed and guilty about the calories.

DESSERTS

Desserts are an enjoyable ending to a good meal. Again plan ahead. Make the decision ahead of time of how to "spend" your calories. Modify your breakfast and lunch that day to accommodate a favorite dessert. When it comes time to ordering dessert think about how hungry you really are, and whether or not you've stuck with your calorie plan for the meal. Many desserts are high in fat, calories, and sugar plus portions tend to be large. This is a good item to split with someone, or everyone, at the table. If eating at a restaurant known for its decadent chocolate cake and chocolate is your thing plan to have it.

Low calorie choices that are a nice finish to a meal are sorbets, sherbets, and fresh fruit. Some restaurants will offer a frozen yogurt or low-fat ice cream. Sometimes a delicious cup of coffee or tea is a satisfying way to end a meal and is all you really need.

PLANNING IS THE KEY

Busy people, especially those who travel are constantly navigating eating situations. Budgeting daily calories is the most creative way to allow for a variety of foods and to accommodate the many different foods and eating styles you may be challenged with. Planning has also become easier with modern technology and cell phones. There is a new app on Android and iphones, and soon Blackberry phones called My Fitness Pal with a database of over 726,000 food and restaurant items, including multicultural foods. By planning in advance, you can eat out sensibly and allow yourself healthy food choices guarding against gaining excessive weight.

Answers to Dining Out Questions:

1. False. With a little planning, you can eat healthy foods when dining out.
2. False. Knowing the calorie level of fast foods allows you to include fast foods in your diet
3. False. Meal layering is helpful in making you feel fuller with less food.
4. True.
5. False.

Guidelines for various types of eating-places are listed below. These tips will provide you with acceptable cooking methods, food items, and suggestions to enhance healthier choices and reduce calories. These guidelines can be used in restaurants or when ordering out.

AMERICAN

Appropriate Methods of Cooking:

Barbequed	Marinated
Blackened Cajun	Mesquite-grilled
Charbroiled	Stir-fried
Grilled	

Acceptable Items:

Barbeque Sauce	Mustard
Cocktail Sauce	Honey mustard

Fajitas	Low-Calorie or Fat-Free Salad Dressing
Jalapenos	Sauteed Onions
Lettuce	Peppers
Tomatoes	Mushrooms
Raw Onions	Spicy Mexican beef or chicken
Watch Out For:	
Alfredo Sauces	Deep fried
Bacon	Golden, lightly or crispy
Bread Crumbs	Guacamole
Butter	Mayonnaise
Cheese	Sausage
Cream	Served in a crispy tortilla shell
Cream Sauces	Sour Cream
Fried Items - battered	"Special Sauces"

Special Requests:

Could you put the salad dressing, sauce on the side?
How is this item prepared?
Could I have a baked potato, salad, or steamed vegetables instead of the French fries?
Could you leave the French fries off the plate?
Could I have whole-wheat bread in place of the croissant?

ASIAN

Appropriate Methods of Cooking:

Baked	Simmered
Barbequed	Steamed

Boiled	Stir-fried
Braised	

Acceptable Items:

Tofu (bean curd)	Fish
Vegetables	Scallops
Shrimp	Chicken
Roast Pork	

Acceptable Items: for those not watching their sodium:

Soy Sauce	Dipping Sauces
Hoisin Sauce	Served on a sizzling platter
Brown Sauce	Slippery White Sauce
Oyster Sauce	Velvet Sauce
Black Bean	Chinese Mustard
Hot and Spicy Tomato	Sweet Sauce
Chili	Light Wine Sauce
Teriyaki Sauce	Lobster Sauce
Miso	Won Ton Soup
Hot and Sour Soup	

Watch Out For:

Duck	Breaded
Cashews	Crispy
Peanuts	Coconut milk or cream
Water Chestnut Flour	Foods fried in lard
Chinese Noodles	Fried bean curd
Served in a bird's nest	Tempura
Sweet and Sour	Agemono
Deep Fried	Katsu
Battered	Pan-fried

Special Requests:

Could you remove the Chinese noodles from the table?
Please remove cashews, almonds, or peanuts, or use a small amount.
Please don't use MSG.
Could you substitute chicken for the duck?
Could you omit or reduce the use of oil or soy sauce?
What type of oil is used in cooking? Could you use peanut oil instead?

FAST FOODS

Appropriate Methods of Cooking:

Baked	Grilled
Acceptable Items or Terms:	
Baked Potato	Onion
French Dip Sandwich	Light
Chili	Reduced Calorie
Grilled Chicken	Fat-free salad dressings
Hamburger (regular, junior, or single)	Low-fat frozen yogurt
Lettuce	Low-fat milk
Tomato	Roast beef

Watch Out For:	
Bacon	Fried Chicken
Cheese (any type)	Mayonnaise-based sauces (tartar)
Cheese Sauce	Salad Dressings
Croissant	Sour Cream
Deluxe anything	

FRENCH FOOD

Appropriate Methods of Cooking:

Broiled	Marinated
Demi-Glace	Poached
En Papillote	Steamed
Grilled	

Acceptable Items:

Au Jus	Sorbet
Bouillabaisse	Vinaigrette

Watch Out For:

Cheese	Pastry
Au Gratin	Confit
Béchamel	Creme Brule
Béarnaise	Creme Fraiche
Beurre Blanc	Crusted
Buttery	Filet of beef Wellington
Caesar Salad	Foie Gras
Canard A l'orange	Gratine
Chateaubriand	Gravy
Coquilles St. Jacques	

Special Requests:

Is this item prepared with oil or cream?

Can it (like butter) be eliminated or reduced?

GREEK FOOD

Appropriate Methods of Cooking:

Baked	Grilled
Steamed	

Acceptable Items:

Soup	Shish-kabob
Mixed Vegetable Salads	Tabbouleh
Rice Stuffed Grape Leaves	Plaki
Pita Bread without butter or oil	Baba Ghanoush
Roasted Eggplant	

Watch Out For:

Pan Fried	Nuts
Phyllo Dough	Olives
Tahini	Anchovies
Tatziki with full-fat yogurt	Falafel
Hummus	Locanico (sausage)
Goat Cheese	Moussaka
Feta	Pastries
Kasseri	

Special Requests:

May I have pita without oil or butter?

If oil or butter is added to this dish, can they be omitted or reduced?

INDIAN FOOD

Appropriate Methods of Cooking:

Tikka	Cooked or marinated in yogurt
Roasted	Tandoori
Marinated	

Acceptable Items:

Vegetables	Papadum
Rice	Matta (pease)
Chapti	Indian spices - curry
Naan	Garam
Tomatoes and Onions	Marsala
Baked leavened bread	Basmati Rice

Watch Out For:

Fried Items	Fritters
Pakora	Rayta with full-fat yogurt
Batter Dipped	Poori
Somosa	Pappadams
Coconut/coconut milk	Ghee
Cream Sauces	Nuts

Special Requests:

Please do not garnish with nuts.
Could I have tea with my meal?
Could you not salt my meal?

ITALIAN FOOD

Appropriate Methods of Cooking:

Marinated	Grilled
Baked	Roasted
Broiled	Sauteed

Acceptable Items:

Polenta	Mushroom Sauce
Pasta with marinara sauce	Seafood
Pasta with red clam sauce	Tomato-based sauces, marinara
Beans	Bolognese
Medallions	Cacciatore
Vinaigrette	Piccata
Tomatoes	Pasta dishes without cheese
Salads	Fresh clam sauce

Watch Out For:

Prosciutto	Stuffed Shells
Cream Sauce	Tortellini
Alfredo Sauce	Olives
Four-cheese	Pepperoni
Fried Eggplant	Salami
Parmesan	Pancetta
Pancetta	Manicotti
Carbonera	Lasagna
Francese	Cannelloni
Milanese	Fried Calamari

Special Requests:

Could you remove the skin from the chicken?

Could you eliminate the olive oil?

Could I have some tomato sauce for the bread?

Could you hold the Parmesan cheese, bacon, olives, pine nuts, sauce?

Could I have the salad dressing on the side?

LATIN AND MEXICAN FOODS

Appropriate Methods of Cooking:

Sauteed	Blackened
Grilled	Baked

Acceptable Items:

Soft tortillas, corn or flour	Salad
Salsa	Rice
Gazpacho	Burritos without cheese
Vegetable	Ceviche (marinated seafood)
Tortilla	Pinto beans, Black beans
Black Bean Soups	Fish Vera Cruz style

Watch Out For:

Fried Items	Chiles Rellenos
Enchiladas	Tacos
Guacamole	Flan
Sour Cream	Sopapillas
Refried beans with lard	Nacho
Cheese quesadillas	Chimichangas
Chorizo (Mexican sausage)	

Special Requests:

Could you cut the cheese in half on this item?

Could you put the guacamole, sour cream, and salad dressing on the side?

Could you take away the chips and salsa?

Is this dish prepared with oil? Can it be eliminated or reduced?

UPSCALE RESTAURANTS

Appropriate Methods of Cooking:

Blackened	Poached
Cajun	Roasted
En Brochette (on skewers)	Steamed
Fruit Sauce	Tomato
Grilled	Garlic
Marinated	Herb Sauces
Mustard sauce, not creamed	

Acceptable Items:

Chipotle Peppers or sauces	Roasted Peppers
Couscous	Salsa - fruit or vegetable
Herbs and spices	Sun-dried tomatoes
Light vinaigrette	Vinegar-balsamic
Polenta	Raspberry
Risotto	

Watch Out For:

Au Gratin	Remoulade Sauce
Bacon	Sausage
Butter	Sour Cream
Special butters or butter sauces	Stroganoff
Casserole cheese (any)	Whipped Cream
Creamed or cream sauces	Wrapped in bacon

Creme Fraiche	Pastry Shell
Hollandaise Sauce	Puffed Pastry
Mornay Sauce	Phyllo Dough

Special Requests:

Could you omit or serve the sauce on the side?
Could you serve the salad dressing on the side?
Could I have some vinegar or lemon for my salad?
Could you bring me butter or sour cream for my baked potato on the side?
Could I have my vegetables steamed rather than sautéed?

AT ALL RESTAURANTS

Acceptable Desserts:

Fresh Fruit	Sherbet
Sorbet	Angel Food Cake

Special Requests:

Before ordering a salad ask the waiter how the salad is prepared.
Reduce or eliminate bacon, cheese, croutons, olives, and mayonnaise-based items from salads.
Ask for salad dressing on the side.
Vinegar and a light amount of oil or lemon are your best choices for salad dressing.

THE SKINNY ON SNACKS

"No man in the world has more courage than the man, who can stop after eating one peanut."

— *Channing Pollock*

Call it what you like: snacking, grazing, noshing; we are a snacking society. There is probably no other country that snacks throughout the day as much as we do. Offices and homes are small convenience stores, making it difficult to avoid the temptation to snack. Some individuals admit to snacking because of boredom or merely because snacks are available, rather than snacking from hunger. For others, snacks are a reward for a tough or busy day at work or dealing with a grouchy boss. One of the drawbacks to frequent snacking is that we tend to forget what it's like to feel hunger. The end result is that we wind up never feeling satisfied and eating too many calories. Not to worry. Snacks can be a great opportunity for some quick nutrition, a pick me up during the day, or even a little guilty pleasure. If you're trying to lose weight, snacks prevent overeating at the next meal, especially if the meal is delayed.

1. **Think before you snack.** Snacking is often impulsive. And visual cues can be the strongest, tempting us to eat even if not hungry. Ask yourself: am I really hungry; when's my next meal;

is there an activity I can do instead of eating? Remember a bite here and there eventually adds up.

2. **Do the math.** Know the calories in the snack you choose, and make sure it fits into your meal plan. Regardless of the nutritional value of a snack, those snack calories are included in your calorie budget. When you exceed your daily allowance, you will gain weight. In fact, if you add 100 calories a day to your current intake with no changes to your activity, you can gain 10 lbs. in one year. It doesn't matter if the snack is an apple or a small Snickers bar. Those extra calories will catch up with you, usually around your waistline.

3. **Limit your choices.** Select a few snacks you enjoy and are within your calorie budget. There's a large variety of snack items to choose from. Many are available in 100-calorie packs. Baggie your favorites: baby carrots, nuts, dried fruit, pretzels, dark chocolate. Planning ahead and allowing for snacks based on their calories and nutrition is the smart way to go.

4. **Kitchen is closed!** Night snacking can pack on the pounds. Most of us eat enough dinner to avoid eating again. There's not much time until bed, so we don't work off those extra calories. If you really want something, try a low-calorie beverage or snack. Keep in mind that snacking will make you stay up longer. If you are tired, go to sleep.

Low carbohydrate, high fiber snacks are a good idea since they will make you feel fuller longer without the extra calories. Fruits and vegetables are good choices. If there is a long time between meals, say more than five hours, a snack with a little protein or fat is a better choice. Fat and protein will stay with you longer, getting you from meal to meal with a minimal amount of hunger. You will then be able to avoid overeating at that next meal.

Avoid using beverages as snacks. Liquids usually don't keep you satisfied for long; you'll find yourself looking for something else to eat an hour or two later. Juices provide very little nutrition and often contain a lot of sugary calories. Read the label before you drink. Remember snacking can be nutritious and easy to incorporate into a healthy eating plan.

SNACKING ON THE GO

The 2015 Scientific Report of the Dietary Guidelines Committee has reported that snacks are becoming more prevalent among millennials (ages 21-38 years). A quarter of millennials are consuming 4 or more snacks daily with a significant increase in snacking than the year before. Millennials are more likely to pick snacks with added nutrition, flavor, and variety. This includes: increased fiber, increased protein, increased vitamins, enhanced energy claims, bold flavor, and variety. They are also more apt to buy organic choices. The majority snack on healthy choices and they prefer that they are ready to eat, smaller portions, convenient packaging, and affordable

Americans overall are now obtaining 25% of their intake from snacks, including children and adolescents. Ninety-six percent of the American public is consuming at least one snack daily. This includes over 2-year-old children. It has been found that 2-3 snacks being consumed daily is more common. In 2014, Americans ate snacks in place of dinner at least one time monthly. Favorite snacks included chips, chocolate, cheese, and fresh fruit. It has been found that only 27% of the population eats the traditional breakfast, lunch, and dinner. The average person eats two meals and three snacks daily. The most common foods consumed at lunch include: cheese, crackers, chips, vegetables, meat proteins, fruit, nuts, and yogurt.

Increased snacking has been associated with decreased protein intake that helps with increased satiety, enhanced weight loss, and maintenance of normal blood sugar levels as a result of improved insulin action. Some researchers are advocating 30% protein at each meal with some protein included at between meal snacks.

Companies are competing rapidly for a piece of the healthy snack market that is projected to be $32 billion by 2025. Restaurants are now offering more smaller menu items and snack companies are creating large snack or small meal offerings. Companies have found that consumers are demanding not only healthier choices but unusual tastes.

Meal scheduling has also changed. Breakfast is often consumed while commuting. Lunches are eaten around meetings and must-do projects. Dinner is looked at as a meal that can be consumed with as little planning, cooking, or cleaning. Rather than people scheduling their busy lives around eating, they now eat around their schedules. This new method of eating is being accommodated at restaurants, drugstores, convenience stores, grocery clubs, supermarkets, and on the internet. For busy people on the go, it's easy to skip meals without ever realizing a meal was missed. You may be caught in a meeting, rushing to make a deadline, or running to drop kids off at school. Despite a hectic schedule, it is important to allow yourself something to eat every four to five hours. This will help avoid feelings of extreme hunger that lead to overeating and weight gain. If there is a refrigerator at work or school, keep a supply of bottled water; diet pop, low-fat yogurt, low-fat cheese, frozen meals, and fruit on hand. A microwave will allow a quick warm up of leftovers, frozen meals, canned soups, popcorn, and hot cereal. Thinking through food needs will avoid visits to the vending machine or take-out restaurants, where choices are high in calories, fat, and cholesterol.

The same holds true when traveling from place to place in the car: keep a supply of healthy snack foods on hand when stopping for a meal isn't possible. A collapsible cooler will provide a cool spot to keep beverages and food safe while traveling. A sport cooler can be purchased at sporting goods stores, Target, Amazon, , or Wal-Mart. They are great for individuals who travel for work. Slip the cooler into a side pocket of a suitcase for use in the hotel room.

When traveling by plane for business or pleasure, make sure to bring a carry-on bag for snacks. As a result of current security measures, most airlines suggest not packing food in suitcases to be checked. Liquid items cannot be brought through the security check-in, but can be purchased once past security.

With today's airline travel, it's easy to get delayed in security checks that allow little time to stop for a meal. And, when there is time, the food is often full of calories and fat. Pre-planning carry-on food for the plane and hotel will eliminate the need for impulse eating. This type of eating is often the result of fatigue, fewer eating choices, and stress. If renting a car, take advantage of the local grocery store rather than the high calorie foods from room service or lobby vending machines. A quick call to the hotel before leaving will provide helpful information about grocery or drug store accessibility, where food and beverages can be purchased for more individual needs.

SNACKS AND CALORIES

SNACKS UNDER 50 CALORIES

Crunchy Snacks	Portion	Calories
Air-popped Popcorn	1 cup	30
Dill Pickle	1 medium	12
Melba Toast	2 pieces	25
Oyster Crackers	10 crackers	33
Saltine Crackers	3 crackers	40
Lupini Beans	1/4 cup	40

Sweet Treats	Portion	Calories
Creamsicle	1 low-calorie	25
Meringue Cookie	1 cookie	35
Flavored sugar-free Gelatin	1 cup	20
Unsweetened Applesauce	1/2 cup	50
Chewing Gum	1 stick	5
Fortune Cookie	1 cookie	15
Gummy Bears	3 bears	20
Hard Candy	1 piece	25
Ice Pop	2 fl. oz. bar	42
Life Savers	4 pieces	36
Lollipop	1 pop	22
Marshmallow	2 large	46

Whipped Topping	2 tablespoons	25
Sugar-free Jelly/Jam	2 teaspoons	30

Fabulous Fruit	Portion	Calories
Apricots	3 medium	50
Blackberries	1/2 cup	37
Cranberries	1 cup	46
Watermelon	1/2 cup	30
Apple	1 small	50
Water packed fruit cocktail	1/2 cup	40
Grapefruit	1/2 medium	37
Orange	1 small	50
Kiwi	1 medium	46
Peach	1 medium	37
Fresh Mixed Fruit	1 cup	50
Grapes	15 grapes	50
Cherries	12 cherries	50
Strawberries	1 cup	50
Banana	1/2 banana	40

SNACKS LESS THAN 100 CALORIES

Great Grains	Portion	Calories
Raisin Bread	1 slice	60
Whole Wheat Bread	1 slice	70
Rye Bread	1 slice	70
Plain Bagel	1/2 medium	88
Chickpea puffs	1 oz.	90

How Cheesy	Portion	Calories
Low-fat string cheese	1 piece	80
Low-fat cottage cheese	1/2 cup	90
Beef Jerky	1 piece	90

Portable Fruits	Portion	Calories
Banana	1/2 banana	53
Blueberries	1 cup	82
Cantaloupe	1 cup, cubed	57
Fruit Salad	1/2 cup	67
Grapes	1 cup	58
Honeydew Melon	1 cup, cubed	60
Mango	1/2 medium	68
Nectarine	1 medium	67
Orange	1 medium	65
Papaya	1/2 medium	58

Something Sweet	Portion	Calories
Rice Krispies	1 bar	90
Special-K bar	1 bar	90
Snack Wells Creme Sandwich	2 cookies	86
Snickers, snack size	1 snack size	52
Twix, snack size	1 snack size	80
3 Musketeers, snack size	3 snack size	75
Licorice	2 pieces	70
Reese's Minis	2 mini cups	84
Candy Corn	10 pieces	51
Sugar-free pudding	1 cup	92
Fig bar	1 bar	53

Gingersnaps	2 cookies	59
Graham crackers	1 large square	60
Wafer - chocolate or vanilla	3 wafers	75
Animal Crackers	5 crackers	56

Hot, Hot, Hot	Portion	Calories
Vegetable Soup	1 cup	72
Chicken Noodle Soup	1 cup	75
Baked Crab Cakes	1 cake	88

Keepin' Cool	Portion	Calories
Fat-free Fudgsicle	1 bar	60
Fat-free Frozen Yogurt	1/2 cup	70
Italian Chocolate Ice	1 scoop	60
Fruit Sorbet	1 scoop	60
Fat-free Ice Cream	1/2 cup	90
Frozen Fruit and Juice Bar	1 bar	75

SNACKS LESS THAN 150 CALORIES

Munch on this...	Portion	Calories
Baked Chips	11 chips	110
Baked Tortilla Chips	20 chips	110
Soy Chips	25 chips	110
Triscuits	7 crackers	120
Sun Chips	10 chips	140
Pretzel Rods	3 rods	110
Veggie Crisps	21 crisps	140
Mini Rice Cakes	15 cakes	120
Wheat Thins	16 thins	150

English Muffin	1 muffin	126
Kale Chips	1 oz.	124
Hippeas	1 oz.	130

Sweet Treats	Portion	Calories
Chex Morning Mix	1 package	130
Quaker Chewy Granola Bar	1 bar	110
Hot Chocolate	1 package	150
Angel Food Cake	1 slice	145
Jelly Beans	10 beans	104
Italian Ice	1/2 cup	120

SNACKS LESS THAN 200 CALORIES

Go Nuts!	Portion	Calories
Almonds	1 oz	166
Cashews	1 oz	170
Macadamia	1 oz	201
Pecans	1 oz	186
Peanuts	1 oz	160
Pistachios	1 oz	156
Walnuts	1 oz	172

The Other Stuff	Portion	Calories
Carnation Instant Breakfast	1 package	200
Tuna, water-packed	1 can	191
Regular Gelatin	1 cup	160
Trail Mix	1/2 cup	173
Nature Valley Granola Bar	1 package (2 bars)	200

Mix it up!	Portion	Calories	Total
Cottage Cheese / Mixed Fruit	1/2 cup / 1 cup	100 / 50	150
Cheese / Crackers	1 oz / 6 crackers	80 / 78	158
Peanut Butter / Whole Wheat Bread	1 tbsp. / 1 slice	78 / 60	138
Peanut Butter / Sugar-free Jelly	1 slice / 2 tsp.	60 / 50	110
Baked Tortilla Chips / Salsa	20 chips / 6 tbsp.	110 / 45	155
Skim Milk / Special-K Bar	1/2 cup / 1 bar	45 / 90	135
Skim Milk / Graham Crackers	1/2 cup / 2 lag squares	45 / 120	165
Veggie Soup / Oyster Crackers	1 cup / 10 crackers	72 / 33	105
Fat-free Yogurt / Grape Nuts Cereal	8 oz / 1 oz	50 / 100	150
Apple / Peanut Butter	1 medium / 1 tbsp.	60 / 87	147

Simple Snack Recipe: Trail Mix

- **Ingredients**

    1 cup Wheat Chex

    1 cup Rice Chex

    1 cup Corn Chex

    1 cup raisins

    1 cup roasted peanuts

- **Directions:** Mix the above together in a large bowl. Three cups of Cheerios can be substituted for the Chex; cranberries can be used in place of the raisins.

- **Makes 10 (½ cup) servings**

  161 calories

  25 grams of carbohydrate

  4 grams of protein

  5 grams of fat

- **Or 15 (1/3 cup) servings**

  100 calories

  17 grams carbohydrate

  3 grams of protein

  2.5 grams fat

POPULAR SNACKS

This chart shows some snack foods that are often available to purchase. Remember that portion sizes are large and can often be split in two.

Miscellaneous Snacks	Size	Calories (g)	Carbohydrate (g)	Protein (g)	Fat (mg)	Cholesterol (mg)	Sodium (g)	Fiber
Einstein Brownie	122 gm.	500	76	4	21	30	280	2
Einstein Chocolate Chip Cookie	113 gm.	600	78	4	28	45	480	2
Einstein Sugar Cookie	113 gm.	610	73	7	32	55	490	1
Einstein Banana Nut Muffin	142 gm.	520	59	9	29	95	430	3
Einstein Chocolate Chip Muffin	57 gm.	240	67	3	13	40	370	0
Einstein Cinnamon Bun with icing	113 gm.	380	64	8	10	0	310	2
Einstein Blueberry Scone	127 gm.	450	64	7	18	55	460	2
Einstein Low-Fat Raspberry Scone	117 gm.	350	74	7	3	25	330	2
Krispy Kreme Doughnut (glazed ring)	52 gm.	200	23	4	11	5	115	2

Einstein Egg Bagel	69 gm.	340	69	11	3	35	510	2
Einstein Cinnamon Swirl Bagel	113 gm.	350	78	11	1	0	490	2
Einstein Power Bagel w. Peanut Butter	117 gm.	750	92	27	34	0	780	7
Einstein Cranberry Bagel	113 gm.	350	78	10	1	0	490	3
Dunkin Donuts Plain Croissant	n/a	290	26	5	18	5	270	<1
Dunkin Donuts Chocolate Chip Muffin	n/a	590	88	9	24	75	560	3
Dunkin Donuts Corn Muffin	n/a	500	78	10	16	80	920	1
Dunkin Donuts Lemon Poppy seed Muffin	n/a	580	94	10	19	85	620	2
Dunkin Donuts Chocolate Bismarck Muffin	n/a	340	50	3	15	0	290	<1
Dunkin Donuts Traditional Doughnut	n/a	240	25	3	15	0	340	<1
Krispy Kreme Chocolate Doughnut (Iced Glazed)	66 gm.	280	36	3	14	>5	75	1
Einstein Chocolate Chip Bagel	113 gm.	370	76	11	3	0	500	3

SECTION 6

EATING ON THE MOVE

SUPER SIZE: LESS IS BEST

*Moderation. Small helpings. Sample a little bit of everything.
These are the secrets of happiness and good health."*

— *Julia Child*

If you find yourself gaining weight, it might be a good time to review your portion sizes. Often, it's not the foods you're eating, but the quantity of food that can get you into trouble and compromise your waistline.

Unfortunately, American portions are becoming a major contributor to weight gain and obesity in this country. Americans are being exposed to a serious case of "Portion Distortion." Many fast-food restaurants offer portions that are from 2 to 8 times greater than portion size from years past. The fast food industry found that by increasing portion sizes, they increase sales and attract new business. "Supersize", "Double Gulp", "Hefty Portions", and "Godzilla sizes" describe some of the menu items offered. A study by Pennsylvania State University showed that when portion sizes are increased, individuals tend to eat more. Surprisingly, the study also found that subjects did not feel any fuller after eating a larger portion than with a smaller one.

Restaurants currently serve six-ounce bagels, although the standard serving size is two ounces. A Dunkin Donuts bagel is about 330 calories compared to a frozen bagel at the grocery store that averages 160 calories. A typical restaurant size steak is eight ounces, when 3-4 ounces is the standard portion size. When pasta is served in a restaurant, patrons are given approximately three-cup servings, when a half-cup serving is the standard portion size.

McDonald's has increased serving sizes of two of the most popular foods served in America. When McDonalds opened, a small serving of French fries contained 210 calories; while today's super-sized order of fries has 540 calories. When a small cola was originally served it contained 16 ounces and 205 calories. Today, a super-sized cola contains 42 ounces and 539 calories. Together these two super-sized items comprise 1079 calories, or more than half the daily energy requirement of most Americans.

Even candy bars have grown larger over the years. Years ago, chocolate candy bars contained 0.6 ounces. Today a small bar weighs in at 1.6 ounces and large bars over 6.0 ounces.

Unfortunately if you eat out frequently your perception of what a portion is can become distorted. Some suggestions for determining proper portions include the following:

Purchase convenient measuring cups for liquids and solids, as well as measuring spoons, to determine portion sizes. Don't use regular cups or spoons that you ordinarily eat from because they are not accurate to measure portions.

Measure out a cup (or a half-cup) of liquid into a glass that you would ordinarily use for your milk or juice.

1. Use measuring cups for foods such as pasta, rice, soup, or mashed potatoes.

2. Place the measuring cup on a flat surface and pour the liquid to the line showing the amount you want. If you hold the cup up in the air, the measurement will not be accurate.

3. Pour the measured amount into an everyday drinking cup and observe the line where the liquid fills. The next time you decide to have a cup of milk, pour the milk into the same

glass. Since you know how full a cup should be, this eliminates the need to physically measure the beverage every time.

4. Allow the same pattern of measuring solid items, such as cereal into a solid measuring cup. After you have measured a cup or half-cup, see where the cereal comes up to on the bowl. Fill the bowl to this point every time you use it.

Buy a modest kitchen scale to measure solid items that cannot be placed in a cup. This will be helpful to measure meats at home.

1. Meats should be weighed after cooking.

2. A rule of thumb is that four ounces of raw meat (without a bone) will weigh approximately three ounces cooked.

3. Five ounces of raw meat with a bone will weigh approximately four ounces cooked.

4. Estimate the weight of the item before you place it on the scale and then check to see how close you come to the actual portion size.

Getting used to how the foods look on your plate will help you when eating out, rather than carrying scales and a measuring cup

1. Ask for a take-out box at the beginning of the meal so that you are not tempted to eat too much.

2. If you can figure out your portions, you will prevent over-eating.

Fill your ice cream scoop or soup ladle with water to see how much it holds.

Purchase individual bags of an item that remind you of a typical portion size to help you restrict your portions.

When you are done with the bag, you are finished eating the item. Try to eat the item slowly, savoring the taste of the food and enjoying it.

After several months check your portion sizes again.

This refresher will allow you to make sure that your perception of your portions has not changed. It will also help keep your waistline in check.

VISUALIZING FOOD PORTIONS

To visualize the size of an item or the size of a measuring tool consider the following guidelines:

Portion Size	Common Household Item
1 tbs. of Peanut Butter or Cream Cheese	Three dice or a walnut
1 oz of Nuts	2 shot glasses
1 oz of Cheese	4 stacked dice
1 slice of Cheese	3½ inch computer disk
1 chunk of Cheese	2 dominos thick
1 medium Potato	Computer Mouse
1 small Banana	Eyeglass Case
1 medium Apple, Pear, or Peach	Tennis Ball
1 cup Broccoli	Light Bulb
1 cup Cereal	Halfway up side of Standard Bowl
½ Chicken Breast, 1 medium Pork Chop, 1 small Hamburger, 1 Fish Fillet	1 deck of cards
1 small Chicken leg or thigh	2 ounces
½ cup Tuna, Cottage Cheese, Pasta	Hockey Puck
½ cup grapes	Light Bulb

Food portions can also be visualized using your hand as a measurement guide.

Portion Size	Hand Measurement
1 Fruit Serving	Finger length diameter
1 tsp. of butter, margarine, or peanut butter	Top half of your thumb
1 cup of Pasta, Cereal, Cooked Vegetables	Fist volume
1 serving of Nuts	1 Handful
1 small Potato	Half of a fist
½ cup of Fruit, Vegetables	Palm of hand
1 serving of Snack Foods	2 Handfuls
4 oz portion of Meat, Fish, Poultry	Palm of hand
1 ounce or 1 tablespoon	Thumb volume
1 teaspoon	Thumb tip

PORTION CONTROL PLATES, BOWLS, AND SCALES

- Portion Control Dinnerware:

  www.preciseportions.com   www.diabetesandmore.com

- Portion Control Bowls & Plates:

  Measure Up Bowl Set, "Measure 2" at Target or Slimware Plate set with 4 plates at bit.ly3ow99AC

- Kitchen Scales, food scales, and cooking scales www.old-willknottscales.com

  PortionMate Measuring Tool at www.portionmate.com

RATE YOUR PLATE WITH THE FOOD GROUPS

It's tough to decide how much food to put on your plate. Let this be your guide! Servings should fit within a 9" plate, or the inner center of a large dinner plate. Go to www.ChooseMyPlate.gov to determine your individual calories and servings. The basic daily requirements to keep in mind are:

Food Group	Daily Requirement	One Serving Size Equal To
Grains	5 oz (½ should be whole grains)	1 slice of bread, 1 cup of cereal ½ cup cooked rice, cooked pasta or cooked cereal
Vegetables	2 cups	1 cup raw or cooked vegetables or vegetable juice 2 cups raw leafy greens counts as 1 cup
Fruit	1½ cups	½ cup dried fruit, 1 cup of fruit 1 small apple (4 oz.) 1 small banana (4 oz.)
Milk	3 cups	1 ½ ounces of natural cheese, 2 ounces processed cheese ¾ cup of plain non-fat yogurt
Meats & Beans	5 oz	1 ounce of meat, poultry or fish ¼ cup cooked dry beans, 1 egg 1 tablespoon of peanut butter ½ ounce nuts or seeds
Oils	5 tsp.	1 teaspoon oil: Canola, Olive, Peanut, 10 Peanuts, 2 teaspoons peanut butter, Mixed nuts, 6 nuts equal 1 teaspoon, Olives: 8 large black olives or 10 large green olives, 1/8 of an avocado

RATE YOUR PLATE USING THE PLATE METHOD

Carbohydrates: Carbohydrates include starchy vegetables (like potatoes) and grains (like whole wheat bread and rice or whole wheat pasta). Carbohydrates at breakfast are greater than for lunch and dinner. Using MyPlate guidelines, choose two servings per meal from grains or starchy vegetables that fit nicely into ¼ of a 9-inch plate for lunch and dinner.

Vegetables: Fill half your plate with non-starchy vegetables, like broccoli, cauliflower, green beans, or carrots. Also, green leafy vegetables, such as salad, counts as a serving of vegetables.

Protein: Keep meat choices to 3-4 ounces twice daily. Meat and Bean choices, shown on the MyPlate guidelines, give ideas for serving sizes for the different types of protein.

Dairy: One cup of milk per meal, or an equivalent, will do it! This requirement ensures there is sufficient calcium in your diet. Dairy also provides protein and carbohydrate.

Fruit: You might find it difficult to eat this much food. If so, save your fruit serving for snacks. Fruit is portable and easy to put in a backpack or briefcase.

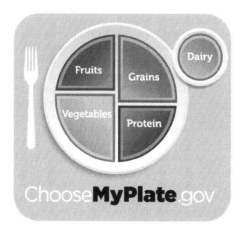

TRAVEL EATING

When a majority of time is spent in the car, running from appointment to appointment, it's helpful to have a method for eating on the road. Many sales representatives (and moms) keep a basket or a shoe box of healthy snacks in the trunk that can be grabbed between appointments. Even if you're short on time, a healthier, and cheaper food choice is as close as the trunk! Collapsible coolers are useful to store items such as diet cold drinks, water, yogurt, low-fat cheese, and sandwiches. Just stick a cold pack in the cooler to keep things cold. These can be purchased at Target, Amazon, Wal-Mart, or sporting goods stores. Collapsible coolers take up little space when folded in the outside pocket of a suitcase. In addition use in the car with Covid 19 having food available for travel is a must to limit time searching for food. Dependence on places for carry-out is also a safer way to obtain food when travel cannot be avoided.

PROTEIN SOURCES ON-THE-GO

Try to keep a source of protein available if you are unable to stop for a quick meal. This would include peanut butter or nuts if a cooler isn't available. With a cooler or refrigerator, foods can include:

- Yogurt
- Cheese, reduced fat
- Lunch Meats, low-fat

- Add: Bottled water, juice bottles, fresh fruit or fruit cups to the above.

When staying at a hotel, try to book hotels that provide a breakfast buffet. These hotels typically offer eggs, bagels, toast, waffles, cereals, fresh fruit, yogurt, juice, and hot breakfast drinks. Take care when selecting food from the buffet, and think through your choices based upon your healthy meal plan. Sitting at a restaurant and ordering a meal will often encourage you to indulge in larger servings which include greater amounts of high calorie, high fat food.

FUELING AT THE GAS STATION

Hard to believe a couple of dietitians are recommending stopping at a gas station for a quick pick-me-up snack or meal? Suffice it to say that gas station foods have changed over the years. Chewing gum, candy bars, donuts, and sodas are still on the first shelf when we walk in the door, but are no longer the only choices to pick from when hungry and on the road. Some gas stations have mini-markets offering a variety of foods and snacks. Grab a nutritious snack or piece together a few items to make a meal that fits into your healthy meal plan.

Use our list of healthy snacks and see what other items you might find when stopping to fuel up!

Healthy options that most gas stations carry

Cereal	Granola Bars
Fat-Free Milk	Deli Sandwiches
Fresh Fruit	Soups (broth-based)
Cheese	Nuts
Whole Grain Crackers and Breads	Bottled Water or Flavored Water

Gas station foods to limit

Regular Soda	Nachos
Candies	Hot Dogs
Sweetened Coffee Drinks	Donuts and Pastries
Sweetened Energy Drinks	Cookies and Brownies
Chips	

AIRPORT TRAVEL

Airline travel is a common part of a busy life. With the stress of post 9/11 and increased security, air travel changed a great deal. Longer time is required at airports to deal with security issues. Based upon cutbacks post 9/11, domestic flights no longer offered meals in flight for most passengers. International flights did offer meals and snacks. More individuals started eating at airports or buying food to eat on the plane.

Airports are beginning to respond to the public's desire for fast and easy meals and quick to grab beverages. Customers are also demanding healthier food choices to meet their nutritional needs. With Covid 19, airport travel has become even more complicated. Some restaurants are offering service with social distancing provided. On planes beverages are limited to water bottles and cans of soda pop and beer. Passengers are buying meals and beverages at the airport before travel. It remains to be seen what will result when a vaccine is widely available to combat this virus. Whether traveling by car, or plane, there are some foods that provide good nutrition, moderate calories, and minimize hunger. Do check the TSA website for what foods are prohibited until after security check, such as beverages.

Travel Food List

Bottled Water	Bagels	Canned light sugar fruits
Diet Pop	Whole Grain Cereal Boxes	Nuts*
Juice Boxes or Cans	Low-Fat Popcorn Bags	Low-Fat Cheeses
Raisins	Pretzels	Fresh Fruit
Dried Fruits	Baked Chips	Sandwiches
Healthy Trail Mixes	Low-Fat Cookies	Rice Cakes
Whole Grain Crackers	Graham Crackers	Nutrition Bars
100-calorie Snack Packs by Nabisco and Kraft	Vegetables with Low-Fat dips	Peanut Butter* (except plane travel)

* Do not carry on planes due to allergy concerns

VACATIONS

For most of us, vacations are viewed as a 'time out' from the busy-ness of our daily routines. A time to kick back, relax, and indulge. Vacations are a reprieve from our fast-paced life. A little planning and you can come home with a stable weight. You might even lose a few pounds. But if you don't, no big deal. Just attempt to get back on track with healthier eating and improved exercise.

We decided to do a little soul searching. Our motto: same rules apply everywhere; all the time. In other words we stick to a meal schedule and continue exercising. In fact, if we think we'll be eating more, we increase our activity. Seeing a city on foot is a great way to build in exercise. We surveyed individuals who don't gain when on vacation and here's what they said:

1. Many individuals look for vacations with built in exercise, walking, hiking, biking, and swimming/snorkeling.

2. Some said they avoid hotels and instead rent a condo, house, or apartment. They can shop and prepare some meals, saving time, money, and calories.

3. On road trips or long flights individuals pack snacks, energy bars, sandwiches.

4. For those staying in hotels, they make sure a refrigerator is available and head to the nearest grocery store for healthy foods/snacks.

5. If it isn't an outdoor vacation, individuals make sure they stay where exercise equipment is available.

6. Individuals staying with relatives try to help plan and shop for meals. This allows them to stay on their diet plan and help out their hosts with the extra costs of having guests.

7. Cruises can become food orgies. Sticking to a meal schedule and avoiding impulse eating is critical. Most increase activity on board ship, signing up for exercise classes, swimming, or walking the ship.

8. Many say they have a drink quota, knowing that calories in a few pina coladas or margaritas add up quickly.

9. When individuals eat all their meals at restaurants, they look for low calorie menus, avoiding fried and breaded foods and opting for fresh simply prepared meals.

10. Many individuals simply split their meals or desserts with their traveling companion.

11. Check your weight before leaving on a vacation and when returning. If there is a scale available, use it.

HOLIDAYS

*"The fondest memories are made gathered
around a table"*

—Unknown

Holidays are a celebration of family, friends, and food. If you've stopped to read this chapter, you may be one that dreads the challenges that accompany holiday eating. For some, extra holiday eating begins around Halloween. For others, it's Thanksgiving that marks the beginning of holiday overeating. We hear it all the time, "I haven't stopped eating since I bought candy for the trick or treaters."

Remember: Eat, drink, and be wary!

Let's face it! The holidays can be stressful, and for some emotionally difficult. Life tends to be busy enough and then suddenly the holidays arrive. Busy days become even busier and our routine takes a backseat to all the demands. Indulging in favorite foods this time of year couldn't be easier or more tempting. Though the 6 to 8 weeks from Halloween to New Year's Day are tough for most of us, we're confident that if you follow some simple rules, do a little calorie budget planning, and have a "no weight gain" motto you'll enter January the same weight as you were before the holidays began.

For starters, be prepared for the party by identifying low calorie items to prepare or bring along.

HOLIDAY SNACKS TO CHOOSE:

- Raw veggies, limiting dips to 2 tablespoons
- 2 Alcoholic beverages for men, 1 alcohol beverage for women
- Wine: one serving is equal to 5 oz.
- Beer: one serving is equal to 12 oz.
- Spirits: one serving is equal to 1 1/2 oz.
- Mixers for Spritzers: Sugar Free carbonated beverages, Water, Seltzer Water

SNACKS TO EAT IN MODERATION:

- Appetizers: don't pile them on the plate; limit the assortment to one small appetizer plate
- Salad dressing and dips, limit to 2 tablespoons
- Fruits, limit to 1/4 cup
- Junk food: limit Chips, Cheese Curls, Corn Chips, etc. to 1/4 cup
- Cookies: choose 1 or 2 small cookies, no more

WATCH THESE GOODIES:

- Chocolate, anything: Cakes, small cookies, fudge are loaded with calories
- Appetizers with Cheese/Meats, including cheese spreads
- Nuts, it's too easy to over indulge
- Junk food: Crackers, Potato Chips, Cheese Curls, Corn Chips, etc.
- Egg Nog, especially with alcohol
- Mixers: Juices, Regular Soda

HELPFUL TIPS TO MAINTAINING WEIGHT THROUGH THE HOLIDAY SEASON:

These are tips we use, and provide our clients, to help maintain weight through the holiday season. Choose a few or all of them. Write them down on a day planner or "to do" list as a consistent reminder of your goals.

1. **Check your weight frequently.** Forget about losing weight during the holidays. Instead, commit to maintaining your weight. By weighing several times a week during the toughest weeks, you'll be able to quickly identify any weight gain and develop a strategy to lose or curb those pounds from adding up.

2. **Stay active.** That's right, don't stop exercising. In fact, if you are eating more calories you'll need to increase your activity/exercise. Try climbing stairs at work or walking during your lunch hour.

3. **Favorite Foods.** Plan to have some of your favorite foods. Deprivation backfires and leads to overeating when your guard is down.

4. **Snack Healthy.** Never go to a party or out to dinner hungry. Eat a high fiber or high protein snack 1-2 hours before the party. These snacks will take the edge off your appetite and make it easier to stick to your plan.

5. **Budget Calories for Alcohol.** Decide ahead of time how much alcohol you will drink. Have a budget of calories to spend on alcohol. Avoid eggnogs and mixed holiday drinks. Instead drink lite beer, champagne, or wine spritzer. Switch to a diet beverage after you've spent your alcohol calories.

6. **Eat the Foods you enjoy.** Eat the foods you enjoy on the main holiday and reduce them during the rest of the season.

Extra pounds come from days of overeating, not from overeating at a single meal or on a single day. Maintain or adjust your usual eating pattern as much as you can on the other days.

7. **Keep Low-Calorie Snacks on Hand.** Make sure you keep low calorie alternatives at home, the workplace, and at parties. Between meal snacking is a challenge during the holidays because of increased availability of high- calorie foods. Always have low calorie choices available to munch on that will keep you away from the infinite parade of cookies and candies.

8. **Keep a Calorie Budget.** Make all your meals meet your calorie budget and save some extra calories for social eating. Every pound on the scale is equal to 3500 extra calories.

9. Fill an appetizer plate with foods you like and move away from the buffet table.

10. **Use an Appetizer Size Plate.** If you fill a smaller plate with the foods you enjoy, and don't go back for seconds, you'll eat less.

11. **Follow the Vacation Eating Guidelines.** If you're staying with family and friends make sure you have foods on hand that fit into your eating style. Bring foods along or take time out to shop when you arrive.

12. **Plan a Time-Out.** Most people complain they overeat when they're tired. Try a short nap, yoga, or a few minutes of quiet time before the party.

Remember, holidays are about family, friends, and fun. Keeping track of calories, staying within a personal calorie budget, and watching your weight will allow you to maintain your weight and still enjoy holiday foods. If you happen to wind up gaining weight after the holidays, get back on track. It is always possible to get back to your program so don't get discouraged!

OFFICE FOOD:
FOOD PUSH AT WORK

Office food seems to be here, there and anywhere and can sabotage healthy eating efforts. Whether it be trying to lose weight or attempting to eat more healthfully, office food does no one any favors.

Office food usually consists of the ever-present candy jar on the desk of your boss, the receptionist, or other well-meaning food providers. It is also the breakfast donuts, cookies, birthday cakes, holiday leftovers, and school fundraiser candy and cookies.

A recent study reported in The International Journal of Obesity showed that individuals at work ate an average of 5.6 pieces of fun-sized candy if placed in a see-through container. If the container was opaque, this was reduced to 3.1 pieces daily. If an individual is sitting close to the candy dish, they add an average of 2.1 pieces daily. Adding only 2 pieces daily of fun-sized candy, without any exercise or dietary change amounts to an increase of 7 pounds each year. Having the candy jar around the office is also quite costly amounting to an annual cost of $546.

How to Avoid The Calorie Tempers and Weight Destroyers

- Bring in healthy snacks that are planned into your diet plan to reduce your urge to splurge.

  Talk to your Human Relations manager about including weight and exercise programs in your company benefits. Encourage them to suggest removal of candy jars and removal of unhealthy food in common areas. Have employees compete for weight loss and exercise program prizes to encourage adherence to programs.

- When sales representatives ask what items they can bring to the office, suggest fruit and other healthy snacks. If they bring in lunch, ask if you can suggest healthy items they can bring or healthy eating-places that they can find healthy choices.

Drink a hot low-calorie beverage to reduce your desire for a high calorie treat. These would include: coffee, tea, low calorie cocoa, or low-calorie apple cider.

Drink a cold low-calorie beverage such as: iced tea, ice water, seltzer water, or diet soda to cut down your consumption of high calorie snacks. Stopping to drink either a cold or hot beverage gives you a chance to stop and think through a high calorie choice.

Reduce office birthday parties to once monthly and suggest a healthy luncheon to your boss in place of high calorie birthday cake.

Remind bosses that stopping by the candy jar, increases time fraternizing, decreases time spent on work, increases employee health risks and obesity, and increases insurance costs.

VENDING MACHINES

We've come a long way from the first vending machine in 215 BC, which dispensed holy water in Egyptian temples. The first vending machine in the U.S. appeared in 1888 and dispensed Tutti-Frutti gum in the subways of New York City. The vending machine of today still offers gum and many more foods that have not much more nutritional value than gum, but a lot more sugar and calories. But change has come, though vending machines haven't completely dispensed with high-calorie, high-sugar snacks. The FDA requires that foods in vending machines have calorie information so consumers can make informed and healthy choices. Many now mark options that are healthier. So, it is easier to make healthier choices. You can sometimes pick your size and even review the nutrition information.

Snacks count as part of your daily meal plan. Rule of thumb: Limit snacks to 100-150 calories each and limit snacks to 2 to 3 per day, depending on your nutrition plan.

Vending machines are designed to tempt those who are hungry and short on time. They can lure us with high calorie, high sugar, high sodium, and high fat choices. Most vending machine users have skipped a meal or don't have other food options available. But the power lies within you to choose the foods that work best for your diet plan and health. The following suggestions can help to reduce your calories from vending machines while still feeding hunger and even cravings.

REDUCING VENDING MACHINE CALORIES

Plan: Buy your own healthy snacks and keep a stash in your desk or office refrigerator. This will save you calories and money.

• Bottled Water	• Low-Fat Cheese Sticks	
• Diet Soda	• Whole Grain Cereal Boxes	• Peanut Butter
• Raisins	• Popcorn (light or no butter)	• Trail Mixes
• Dried Fruits	• Graham Crackers	• Whole Grain Crackers
• Nuts	• Low-Fat Cookies	• Fresh Fruits/Vegetables
• Rice Cakes	• Fruit Cups	• Low-Fat Yogurt

Label: Keep snacks in a baggie and label with your name to discourage food thieves.

Prepare Choices: Study the items found in the vending machine to find the healthy snacks and choose these snacks when the urge hits. This will cut down on impulse buys.

Rewards: Compare the cost of the healthy choices from the vending machine with the cost of the same items purchased at the store.

Put your savings into a jar and reward yourself with special, nonfood treats such as movie tickets, a manicure, or a massage.

HEALTHY VENDING MACHINE SNACKS:

• Bottled Water	• Low-Fat Milk	• Whole Grain Cereal Bars
• Diet Soda	• Pretzels	• Turkey, Ham, Chicken Sandwiches
• Canned Fruit	• Low-fat popcorn	• Tea (unsweetened or diet)
• Dried Fruits	• Nuts	• Coffee, Plain
• Fresh Fruit	• Canned Fruit	• Hard-cooked eggs

UNHEALTHY VENDING MACHINE SNACKS:

• Most cookies	• Snack Cakes	• Sausage Meats/Jerky (high sodium)
• Candy	• Cupcakes	• Cheese Crackers
• Chips	• Pork Rinds	• Regular Soda
• High-fat Crackers	• Sweetened Tea	• Fruit Punch or Lemonade

BEVERAGES: CONSUMED FOR THE TASTE OF THEM

Sugar-sweetened beverage consumption has doubled in the last twenty years. It has been estimated that 20% of the calories consumed in the American diet are from beverages. But beverages don't provide the sense of fullness that food does. This lack of satiety can lead to a large number of calories consumed that don't provide much in the way or nutrition. Plus, portion sizes have increased dramatically. At fast food restaurants or convenience stores, beverages can be a quart -- 32 ounces – or more. That one drink can add 480 calories to your daily intake.

Recent beverage recommendations were made by a panel of nutritionists in the March 8, 2006 issue of *American Journal of Clinical Nutrition*.

RECOMMEND BEVERAGE INTAKE FOR ADULTS:

- Unsweetened tea or coffee: up to 40 oz
- Sugar-sweetened soda, juice, or drinks: up to 8 oz
- Low-fat or skim milk and soy beverages: up to 16 oz
- Diet soda and other non-caloric drinks: up to 32 oz
- Alcoholic beverages: one drink for women daily and two drinks for men daily. A drink equals 12 oz beer, 5 oz wine, or 1.5 oz spirits.

Americans are encouraged to drink primarily water and limit caloric beverages. Beverages should make up only 10% to 14% of daily calories. Beverages are often overlooked when individuals are working on managing calories and weight. Soda and juice may make it into the conversation, but creamer in coffee, sports drinks and alcoholic drinks may be overlooked. Is it time for you to rethink your drink?

SMOOTHIES:
BLENDED, NOT STIRRED

Smoothies are a popular breakfast substitute. They are fast to make and tasty and fast to drink. Smoothies can also be an easy way to add fruits and vegetables to your diet.

Smoothies are nutrient dense and are a concentrated sources of cancer fighting phytonutrients. The charts below show various ingredients you can add to your smoothie. Make sure you do not exceed 250-500 calories. This ensures you are not turning a healthy meal substitute into a high calorie, high sugar snack.

Making a Healthy Smoothie

The best way to make a smoothie is to choose ingredients out of the 6 columns and puree in a blender. You may have to experiment with the ingredients to come up with the best consistency and flavor for you. Please note that the ingredients noted are what many individuals have found to be tasty and depend on individual preference.

Some Smoothie Tips

- Frozen fruit eliminates the need for ice.
- If using fresh fruit, decrease the amount of liquid used.
- To get a smooth green smoothie, blend the leafy greens first in stages to avoid chunks of leafy greens.
- After blending the leafy greens, add liquid and fruit.

- Do not defrost frozen leafy greens. Add frozen greens directly to the blender.

- Smoothie can be made the night before, but use an airtight lid to keep as fresh as possible. Give it a shake before drinking.

- Remember that greens added overnight can give the smoothie a bitter taste. Blend the greens separately in the morning and then add to smoothie mix.

- Add ginger or cinnamon for taste.

Fruit

(Fresh or Frozen)	Amount	Calories
Berries	1 cup	84
Banana	1 cup	134
Mango	½ cup	99
Peach	½ cup	60
Pineapple	½ cup	37

*Cut each fruit into slices

Vegetables	Amount	Calories
Carrots	½ c. chopped	26
Spinach	½ c. chopped	3
Kale	½ c. chopped	17

Protein	Amount	Calories	grams Protein
Whey Powder	1 scoop	103	17
Casein Powder	1 scoop	150	25
Cottage Cheese	¾ cup	134	20
Tofu	3 ounces	52	6
Liquid	Amount	Calories	grams Protein
Cold Water	1 cup	0	0
Yogurt	1 cup	80-100	12
Coconut Water	1 cup	45	2

Skim milk	1 cup	80	8
Soy Milk	1 cup	127	11
Almond Milk	1 cup	40	1.5
Orange Juice	1 cup	120	0
Ice	3 cubes	0	0

Fat	Amount	Calories	grams Fat
Almonds	2 tbs.	103	9
Peanut Butter	1 tbs.	95	8
Almond Butter	1 tbs.	95	8
Flaxseed Oil	1 tbs.	120	14
Avocado	$\frac{1}{2}$	161	15

Additional Add-ons	Amount	Calories
Chia Seeds	1 tbs.	60
Flaxseed meal	1 tbs.	30
Cacao nibs	1 tbs.	65
Cocoa powder	1 tbs.	12
Uncooked oats	$\frac{1}{2}$ cup	145

Smoothie Recipes

Snack Smoothie

> Add 1 cup of frozen berries and 1 cup 80-100 calorie yogurt. Blend together.

> Calories= approximately 142

Breakfast Smoothie

> Add 1 cup of frozen banana, 1 cup 80-100 calorie yogurt, 1 tbs. of peanut or almond butter. Blend together.

> Calories= approximately 329

Breakfast Smoothie

Add ½ cup frozen mango, ½ cup frozen pineapple, 1 cup 80-100 calorie yogurt,

½ cup chopped spinach or kale, and 2 tbs. ground flaxseed meal. Blend together.

Calories= approximately 293

Breakfast Smoothie

Ginger Orange Green Smoothie

Add ½ cup spinach, 1 cup frozen banana, 1 cup orange juice, 1 tbs. chia seeds, and 1 tbs. of ginger.

Blend together.

Calories= approximately 317

Higher Calorie Smoothie

Add 1 cup whole milk, 1 package of Carnation Instant Breakfast Vanilla or 1 scoop of protein powder, 1 cup frozen banana and ½ cup uncooked oats. Blend together. Add cinnamon to taste.

Calories= approximately 363 calorie

CAFFEINE: NO EXPRESSO, DEPRESSO

"The morning coffee has an exhilaration about it which the cheering influence of the afternoon or evening tea cannot be expected to reproduce"

— Oliver Wendall Holmes

Caffeine Questions: Test your knowledge by answering True or False to the questions below.

1. Coffee is the highest caffeine-containing food product.
2. Caffeine is additive..
3. I can use caffeine to lose weight because it decreases my appetite.
4. There are no adverse effects to consuming caffeine products.
5. The recommended intake of caffeine is less than 300 mg per day.

Whether it's a morning cup of coffee or an afternoon pick me up, most of us can't imagine starting our day without a cup of coffee. Coffee is the highest caffeine- containing food used in the American diet. Other items include: tea, cola, energy drinks, chocolate, and some prescription and non-prescription drugs.

FACTS ABOUT CAFFEINE

Caffeine is the most commonly used stimulant in the world found in a variety of plants. It stimulates the nervous system and boosts human performance by speeding up reaction times and increasing alertness. Although caffeine is not addictive, it can be habit forming. When stopped abruptly, individuals can experience headaches, irritability, fatigue, and/or drowsiness.

Once caffeine is taken, it is absorbed into the blood and body tissues in approximately 45 minutes. The peak concentration of caffeine occurs within the first 15-20 minutes after ingestion. Caffeine's half -life is about 4 hours but it is reduced or extended in various groups including pregnant women, children, smokers, and those with liver disease.

Its half-life is influenced by how fast it is metabolized. Smoking, broccoli and other cruciferous vegetables increase metabolism of caffeine. It is increased with alcohol consumption, grapefruit juice, pregnancy, and childhood. As a result of its increased metabolism in pregnant women, the FDA has recommended that pregnant women drink no more than 2 (8 ounce) cups of coffee daily.

Children tend to have very low intakes of caffeine that is mostly derived from cocoa based items, soft drinks, and energy drinks. Very few children drink coffee before the age of 14.

In children and adolescents with lower body weights, caffeine may present a problem with falling asleep and effecting the duration of sleep if taken close to bedtime.

For adolescents, caffeine consumption may benefit athletes in sports performance and also increasing cognitive function.

The FDA has stated that decaffeinated coffee is safe. Ethyl Acetate that can be harmful in large amounts is used in very small amounts in decaffeinated coffee and is considered safe.

Steven L. Miller, a neuroscientist has found that drinking coffee between 9:00-11:00AM and 1:00-5:00PM are the best times for caffeine efficiency. These times are associated with high levels of cortisol coming down resulting in decreased alertness. After lunch is a good time for coffee because of the natural low we feel after lunch and the lowering of cortisol levels.

During peak cortisol producing times, Miller suggests avoiding caffeine. These times include: 8-9AM, 12:00PM-1PM, and 5:30PM-6:30PM.

A new app is being developed by the Montana State University Tech Link Center that will allow personalized scheduling for caffeine dosing. It is predicted to be out this year.

Positive Caffeine Effects

- Enhances mood and alertness
- Helps in weight loss and weight maintenance
- Reduces risk of Type II Diabetes
- Increases energy during work-outs and athletic competition
- Reduces risk of cancer including colorectal, liver, kidney, melanoma, oral/ pancreatic, and bladder
- Effective in reducing Alzheimer's Disease, Parkinson's Disease, liver disease, and bone disease

Some of the research conducted on caffeine consumption show a number of positive results for its inclusion. A Harvard study showed that consuming coffee daily can reduce Type II diabetes. When more than 6 cups of coffee were consumed daily, men's diabetes risk was reduced by 54% and women's risk by 30% compared to non-coffee drinkers.

Tomas DePaulis, a Ph.D. research scientist at Vanderbilt University Institute, has done a number of coffee studies. He has found that regular coffee drinkers are 80% less likely to develop Parkinson's disease. Other research has shown that consuming at least 2 cups of coffee daily can reduce colon cancer risk by 25%, liver cirrhosis by 80%, and gallstones by 50%.

The American Heart Association found that adults drinking one cup of caffeinated coffee daily boosted their blood flow compared to when drinking decaffeinated. Researchers looked at finger blood flow since this relates to how well the smallest blood vessels work. Those with poor blood flow in their small blood vessels show an increased risk of heart attack, heart disease, and stroke. Researchers suspect that caffeine opens up the blood vessels and has anti-inflammatory properties.

A study from Harvard School of Public Health reviewed data from three large studies of nearly 200,000 adults. They found that the risk of suicide was reduced for adults drinking two to four cups of caffeinated coffee compared to those drinking decaffeinated coffee. Researchers believe that caffeine boosts neurotransmitters in the brain like serotonin, dopamine, and noradrenalin that act as mild anti- depressants.

The Journal of Epidemiology reported that people who drank at least one cup of coffee daily reduced throat cancer or mouth cancer by 20% with one to two cups of caffeinated coffee daily and by 50% when consuming more than four cups daily versus those drinking none.

Evidence has also shown that coffee may reduce asthma symptoms, stop headaches, elevate mood, and prevent cavities. The compound that gives coffee its aroma and bitter taste has been found to be responsible for its antibacterial and adhesive properties that prevent dental cavities from forming.

Research reported on August 25, 2020, has cautioned pregnant women to cut out coffee and caffeine containing products. Dr. Zahn Vice President of Practice Activities of the American College of Obstetrics and Gynecology (ACOG) and Gynecology has stated that ACOG sees no need to alter its recommendations for use of caffeine during pregnancy. "Our guidance remains that moderate caffeine consumption, less than 200 mg per day, does not appear to be a major contributing factor in miscarriage or preterm birth," Zahn has stated. Research will continue to determine what the recommendation should be for pregnant women so that an international consensus can be established.

Negative Caffeine Concerns

It can:

- Reduce fine motor coordination
- Cause insomnia dependent on the individual
- Can result in headaches, nervousness, dizziness, irritability, or anxiety
- Increased heartbeat
- Cause excessive urination
- Result in upset stomach if taken on an empty stomach
- Cause stomach discomfort due to caffeine's production of acid

The 2015 Dietary Guidelines state, "Strong and Consistent evidence show that coffee consumption between 3-5 cups daily or up to 400 mg daily is not associated with increased risk of chronic diseases such as cardiovascular disease (CVD), cancer, and premature death in adults.

DANGERS OF ENERGY DRINKS

The trend of using energy drinks by young people to boost their energy can be problematic. In November 2011, the Federal Substance Abuse and Mental Health Services Department reported that since 2005, emergency room visits for energy drink use has risen ten-fold in the U.S. Forty-four percent of young adults are also combining the use of energy drinks with alcohol and drugs. Kids are coming into the emergency room with heart palpitations, light-headedness, dizziness, headaches, and feeling faint. Young adults may be placing themselves at risk due to the fact that energy drinks may contain three times the caffeine as colas. Mixing energy drinks with booze is particularly dangerous. This is because the caffeine keeps them awake, allowing them to drink much more alcohol. Dr. Tom Scaletta, the director of Edward's Hospital emergency room in Naperville, IL, finds these young adults unarousable due to the amount of alcohol they've drank.

Many people are unaware of the amount of caffeine they consume daily. It is important to recognize the adverse effects of caffeine and adjust your intake accordingly. Caffeine should be avoided completely if health concerns are an issue and always consult with your physician and dietitian to decide your specific needs.

If you need to reduce your caffeine intake due to undesirable symptoms or health reasons, check the chart below for suggestions. Always check with your physician or dietitian to make a plan specific to your needs. As with all foods, moderation is the key.

SUGGESTIONS FOR REDUCING CAFFEINE INTAKE:

- Limit caffeine intake to no more than 200-300 mg each day, about two cups of coffee (8 ounces each).
- Drink half decaffeinated coffee or colas and half regular coffee or colas.
- Substitute with decaffeinated beverages and herbal teas.
- Eat meals at regular times with no more than four hours between each meal.
- Get adequate sleep.
- Establish a regular exercise schedule. Run, walk, bike, swim, do yoga, meditate.
- Choose healthier foods. Fatty foods and alcohol can make you drag, causing you to respond with a caffeinated beverage.

CAFFEINE CONTENT IN FOODS AND DRUGS

Over the Counter Drugs	Serving Size	Caffeine (mg)
NoDoz, maximum strength; Vivarin	1 tablet	200
Excedrin	2 tablets	130
NoDoz, regular strength	1 tablet	100
Anacin	2 tablets	64

Juice	Serving Size	Caffeine (mg)
Juiced	10 oz	60
Java Juice	12 oz	90

Coffee	Serving Size	Caffeine (mg)
Coffee, brewed	8 oz	135
Coffee, expresso	2 oz	120
General Foods International Coffee, Orange Cappuccino	8 oz	102
Coffee, instant	8 oz	95
Coffee, instant decaffeinated	8 oz	2
General Foods International Coffee, Cafe Vienna	8 oz	90
Maxwell House Cappuccino, Mocha	8 oz	60 - 65
General Foods International Coffee, Swiss Mocha	8 oz	55
Maxwell House Cappuccino, French Vanilla or Irish Cream	8 oz	45 - 50
Maxwell House Cappuccino, Amaretto	8 oz	25 - 30
General Foods International Coffee, Viennese Chocolate Cafe	8 oz	26

Maxwell House Cappuccino, decaffeinated	8 oz	1 - 5
Coffee, decaffeinated	8 oz	5

Tea	Serving Size	Caffeine (mg)
Celestial Seasonings Iced Lemon Ginseng Tea	16 oz	100
Bigelow Raspberry Royale Tea	8 oz	83
Tea, leaf or bag	8 oz	50
Iced Tea	12 oz	70
Mint Tea	8 oz	50
Oolong Tea	8 oz	40
Orange and Spice	8 oz	45
Snapple Iced Tea, all varieties	16 oz	42
Lipton Natural Brew Iced Tea Mix, unsweetened	8 oz	25 - 45
Lipton Tea	8 oz	35 - 40
Lipton Iced Tea, assorted varieties	16 oz	18 - 40
Lipton Natural Brew Iced Tea Mix, sweetened	8 oz	15 - 35
Nestea Pure Sweetened Iced Tea	16 oz	34
Tea, green	8 oz	30

Tea (continued)	Serving Size	Caffeine (mg)
Arizona Iced Tea, assorted varieties	16 oz	15 - 30
Lipton Soothing Moments Blackberry Tea	8 oz	25
Nestea Pure Lemon Sweetened Iced Tea	16 oz	22
Tea, instant	8 oz	15

Lipton Natural Brew Iced Tea Mix, diet	8 oz	10 - 15
Lipton Natural Brew Iced Tea Mix, decaffeinated	8 oz	< 5
Celestial Seasonings Herbal Tea, all varieties	8 oz	0
Celestial Seasonings Herbal Tea, bottled	16 oz	0
Lipton Soothing Moments Peppermint Tea	8 oz	0

Soft Drinks	Serving Size	Caffeine (mg)
Josta	12 oz	58
Mountain Dew	12 oz	55.5
Surge	12 oz	52.5
Diet Coke	12 oz	46.5
Coca-Cola classic	12 oz	34.5
Dr. Pepper, regular or diet	12 oz	42
Squirt Ruby Red	12 oz	90
Mello Yellow	12 oz	53
Sunkist Orange Soda	12 oz	42
Pepsi-Cola	12 oz	37.5
Barqs Root Beer	12 oz	22.5
7-up or Diet 7-up	12 oz	0
Barqs Diet Root Beer	12 oz	0
Caffeine-free Coca-Cola or Diet Coke	12 oz	0
Caffeine-free Pepsi-Cola or Diet Pepsi	12 oz	0
Minute Maid Orange Soda	12 oz	0
Mug Root Beer	12 oz	0
Sprite or Diet Sprite	12 oz	0

Energy Drinks	Serving Size	Caffeine (mg)
Red Bull	8.3 oz	80
Amp	16 oz	143
Full Throttle Energy	16 oz	144
Rockstar	16 oz	160

Caffeinated Water	Serving Size	Caffeine (mg)
Java Water	1/2 liter	125
Krank 20	1/2 liter	100
Aqua Blast	1/2 liter	90
Water Joe	1/2 liter	60 - 70
Aqua Java	1/2 liter	50 - 60

Caffeinated Water	Serving Size	Caffeine (mg)
Ben & Jerry's No Fat Coffee Fudge Frozen Yogurt	1 cup	85
Starbucks Coffee Ice Cream, assorted flavors	1 cup	40 - 60
Haagen-Dazs Coffee Ice Cream	1 cup	58
Haagen-Dazs Coffee Frozen Yogurt, fat-free	1 cup	40
Haagen-Dazs Coffee Frozen Yogurt, low-fat	1 cup	30
Starbucks Frappuccino Bar	1 bar (2.5 oz)	15
Healthy Choice Cappuccino Chocolate Chunk or Cappuccino Mocha Fudge Ice Cream	1 cup	8

Yogurt	Serving Size	Caffeine (mg)
Dannon Coffee Yogurt	8 oz	45
Yoplait Cafe Au Lait Yogurt	6 oz	5
Dannon Light Cappuccino Yogurt	8 oz	< 1
Stonyfield Farm Cappuccino Yogurt	8 oz	0

Chocolates and Candies	Serving Size	Caffeine (mg)
Hershey's Special Dark Chocolate Bar	1 bar	31
Perugina Milk Chocolate Bar with Cappuccino Filling	1/3 bar	24
Hershey Bar, milk chocolate	1 bar	10
Coffee Nips, hard candy	2 pieces	6
Cocoa or Hot Chocolate	8 oz	5
Chocolate Chips	1 cup	104

Sources for Table:

Serving sizes are based on commonly eaten portions, pharmaceutical instructions, or the amount of the leading-selling container size. For example, beverages sold in 16-ounce or half-liter bottles were counted as one serving.

National Coffee Association, National Soft Drink Association, Tea Council of the USA, and information provided by food, beverage, and pharmaceutical companies and J.J.

Barone, H.R. Roberts (1996) "Caffeine Consumption." Food Chemistry and Toxicology, vol. 34, pp. 119-129.

Bowes &Church's Food Values of Portions Commonly Used. 17th Edition, J.B. Lippincott Company, 1994, pg. 381

Answers to Caffeine Questions:

1. True.
2. False. Caffeine is not addictive but it is habit forming.
3. True. Caffeine has been found to help with weight loss and weight maintenance.
4. False. The adverse effects of caffeine are irritability, tiredness, anxiety, hunger, and inability to focus.
5. True.

ALCOHOL

"Drink the first. Sip the second slowly. Skip the third."

— Knute Rockne

lcohol Questions: Test your knowledge by answering True or False to the questions below.

1. Both men and women should only consume 1 drink or fewer a day.
2. A serving of an alcoholic drink is 12 oz of beer, 5 oz of wine, or 1 ½ oz of spirits.
3. I do not have to worry about drinking alcohol when trying to lose weight because alcohol does not have many calories.
4. Alcohol can compromise a person's decision making by lowering the blood sugar level and dulling the senses.
5. Alcohol consumption during the cocktail hour can increase your consumption of food when the meal is served.
6. Alcohol has been implicated in some research studies for increasing cancer risk.

Whether you're celebrating an event, enjoying a before-dinner cocktail, or sipping a great Merlot, know the facts about alcohol.

Alcoholic beverages are a common part of our social and business lives. Unfortunately, alcohol supplies many empty calories and provides little nutrition. Excess alcohol can damage the body, especially the liver and brain. The latest research recommends no more than one drink per day for men and women. One serving is equal to 12 oz of beer, 5 oz of wine, or 1 ½ oz of spirits. Women physiologically metabolize alcohol less efficiently than men. Men have 20 to 30 percent more water in their systems diluting the alcohol ingested.

THE EFFECTS

The effects of alcohol are many and knowing them is important if you consume alcohol on a regular basis. Alcohol metabolism begins in the stomach and continues into the liver, where alcohol is metabolized. However, if alcohol consumption is too high and too fast for the liver to keep up, the alcohol will enter the blood system. This is when the adverse effects occur on many cells, in particular brain cells.

Alcohol is a diuretic and like any diuretic can cause dehydration if taken in large amounts. Alcohol can also irritate the stomach, making it a good idea to eat when drinking.

Alcohol ingestion causes a lowering of blood sugar levels, also known as hypoglycemia. It takes only two ounces of alcohol to produce hypoglycemia in a fasted person, which will also reduce inhibitions. The combination of low blood sugar and alcohol consumption can make us hungrier as well. When consuming cocktails, munching on appetizers and enjoying the company of others, it is common to lose track of what we eat and drink causing us to overdo it. Alcohol is relatively high in calories; there are 7 calories per gram of alcohol and 20 calories per ounce. If those extra calories are not burned up in the form of exercise, they are stored as fat. Although the cocktail hour is a common American custom, it is far better to eat before drinking to avoid the effects of alcohol consumption. These effects include:

increased hunger, increased consumption of food, and increased storage of fat.

Also know that how quickly you down that drink affects the rate at which alcohol is absorbed into your bloodstream, and how intoxicated you will feel. A martini sipped over an hour will have the same effect as a glass of wine drunk in a half hour. Research also showed that individuals who had a bubbly or carbonated drink may feel the effects of alcohol sooner rather than later.

THE ADVANTAGES

Moderate drinking may:

1. Lower the risk of heart disease, sudden heart attack, and death from cardiovascular disease
2. Lower the risk of stroke
3. Reduce incidence of diabetes
4. Increase gallstones

The good news is that some research has shown that moderate intake of beer, wine, or spirits can aid in protecting the heart. This happens because alcohol can reduce the "stickiness" of blood that can contribute to blood clots. Another study showed that individuals who had one to six drinks a week had higher levels of HDL cholesterol, the "good" cholesterol.

Red wine has a phytochemical called resveratrol. Studies have shown that resveratrol prevents clotting and plaque formation in the arteries. Red wine contains more resveratrol than white wine. The amount of resveratrol in wine depends upon the amount of time the skin of the grape is left on while making the wine. In the case of white wine, the skin is removed before the fermentation so it has a lower concentration. Resveratrol can also be found in grape juice (the purple grape juice), red grapes, cocoa, dark chocolate, peanuts, blueberries, mulberries, and is also sold as a supplement.

In July 2014, research studies were reported in JAMA (Journal of the Medical Association) and BMJ (British Medical Journal) that questioned the effectiveness of resveratrol with heart health. There has been much criticism about the studies and the media's reaction to them. More studies need to be done before the effectiveness of resveratrol and improvement of heart health can be assured.

THE DISADVANTAGES

Excessive drinking may result in:

- Liver disease including cirrhosis, liver failure requiring liver transplantation, and liver cancer.
- A 50% increase in the risk of hypertension, was reported in a study from 2004 by the State University of New York at Buffalo
- Drinking one alcoholic beverage a day increased a woman's breast cancer risk by 10 to 30%, according to American Cancer Society Senior Epidemiologist Heather Spencer Feigelson, PhD
- Risk of heart failure and dementia
- Alcohol poisoning that can be fatal if a lot of alcohol is taken over a short period of time.
- Higher risk of colon cancer
- Risk of injury including accidents due to drunk driving, falls, homicides,
- Suicides, and problems with social and family relationships
- Development of a permanent red face due to alcohol dilating blood vessels that stretch the capillaries in your face
- Risk to the development of the fetus called Fetal Alcohol Syndrome that leads to problems with brain development and possible developmental problems.

Drunkorexia

College students understand the importance of never drinking on an empty stomach due to risk of getting inebriated too quickly. Despite this knowledge, many college students refuse to eat anything all day before drinking. This is a concern because it has been estimated that approximately 60 per cent of college students drink alcohol.

This practice is called drunkorexia or alcoholemia and it is a combination of an eating disorder and alcoholism that is a very dangerous combination. This practice can also include excessive exercising or purging before excess alcohol consumption. This condition is part of the student's desire to be the life of the party along with staying extremely thin. These individuals drink a huge amount of alcohol in a short period of time. The danger lies in the fact that the alcohol is absorbed rapidly with no food in the stomach. This leads to inebriation, vomiting, passing out, or alcohol poisoning. This situation becomes problematic because it can lead to accidents getting home, sexual assault, fights, blackouts, and hangovers affecting school performance.

Prioritizing alcohol over healthy nutrition can lead to nutritional deficiencies such as B vitamins, calcium, magnesium, protein, and fiber. This condition is more common than once thought. Two reports showed that 81 percent of student drinkers had tried this practice and the other showed that as high as 81 percent of students drinking heavily had tried this.

Tavis Glassman, professor of health education and public health at University of Toledo in Ohio is pushing along with other colleagues to add the diagnosis drunkorexia to the Diagnostic and Statistical Manuel of Mental Disorders (DSM). This would be a subheading under the Other Specified Feeding and Eating Disorders. This is important because it will allow payment for services.

Colleges are beginning to add programs on body image, dangers of drunkorexia, and ways to improve their health and their bodies.

Students are also encouraged to support their friends and guide them in getting help for this dangerous practice. More and more campuses are providing services to help students to discontinue this harmful practice.

HANGOVER HELP

Hangovers are no fun, but there are a number of things you can do to feel better.

1. Sip a glass of water between drinks to avoid dehydration.
2. Drink a glass of water before bed and in the morning upon awakening. Adding lemon, that is alkalinic, will help neutralize the acid in the stomach.
3. Stay clear of fatty and fried foods, which will further tax the liver.
4. Avoid anti-hangover products that have not undergone clinical studies to prove effectiveness and safety.
5. If you are dehydrated, eat foods high in salt and potassium. Try some salty soup, fruit, or fruit juices. Orange and grapefruit juice and bananas are good sources of potassium.
6. Avoid spicy foods with an upset stomach.
7. Try Abbott's Pedialyte Sparkling Rush Powdered Drink Mix. This product supplies the necessary electrolytes and carbohydrate for optimal rehydration. It is also helpful for relieving an upset stomach. It is most effective when taken before going to bed.
8. Drink coconut water that is also a good source of sodium and potassium helping with rehydration.
9. Avoid drinks with high levels of congeners

DRINKS WITH HIGH LEVELS OF CONGENERS:

- Bourbon
- Brandy
- Dark-colored beers and beers with a high alcohol content
- Red Wine
- Scotch
- Tequila

THE CULPRIT

Congeners are chemicals found in dark colored drinks. They add color and flavor and are more apt to cause a hangover. Light colored beverages, such as vodka, gin, and light beers are less likely to cause hangover effects than dark colored drinks.

Although health professionals and the government has urged drinking less through the years, the millennials are now taking action. They are starting a trend towards mindful drinking or total avoidance. Last year, alcohol consumption dropped. Beer consumption dropped even more. As a group they are very concerned about their health and they are favoring experiences rather than spending evenings drinking with friends. Covid however; has led to more drinking among all age groups.

With the legalization of marijuana on the horizon, those in the liquor business anticipate even lower volumes consumed. Beer makers are increasing their production of non-alcoholic beers and increasing craft beers. Hard liquor companies are also starting to produce drinks with less calories and less alcohols. A new product Ketel-One has fewer calories than vodka and 40% less calories. They are also readier to drink alcoholic beverages that are seltzer based with lower alcohol, sugar, and calorie contents. Another millennial alcohol favorite is alcopops. They are alcoholic sodas that are favorites with younger drinkers.

Guinness maker Diageo released the Smirnoff Ice Smash. It is fruit flavored and 8 % alcohol by volume. Although millennials are choosing more healthy choices, Miller Lite launched a sixth flavor of an 8% alcohol alcopop called Spiked Tropic Storm. It has been a very solid seller. They also released another alcopop called Redd's Wicked. The alcopops with more alcohol than beer appear popular on occasions where millennials are not worrying about alcohol, sugar, or calorie contents.

SIMPLE TIPS FOR ALCOHOL USE:

- Limit alcohol consumption to one alcohol serving for women and two for men daily.
- Consume a snack such as fruit or crackers before you drink to prevent low blood sugar that can cause hunger and over-eating.
- Limit drinks that contain large quantities of sugar such as liqueurs, sweet wines, fruit juice, soda pop, tonic water, or drink mixes.
- Sugar-free soda pop or drink mixes and soda water are healthier choices and reduce calories and sugar significantly.
- Light beer could be preferable to regular beer and ale, because it has lower calories, carbohydrate, and alcohol. But the amount consumed is important to keep in mind.
- Remember to count the calories from alcohol as part of your daily intake.
- Cut down your use of alcohol by drinking a diet drink or water between each alcoholic beverage consumed.
- Switch to a Shirley Temple or "mocktail" after a drink or two; a spritzer with a small amount of juice is a good substitute.
- Drink your beverages slowly.

Answers to Alcohol Questions:

1. False. Men can drink 2 drinks per day
2. True
3. False. Alcohol provides 7 calories per gram of ethanol. This is more energy than what carbohydrates and protein provide.
4. True
5. True
6. True

DIGESTING THE BAR FACTS

Energy bars are convenient, small, with little clean up required. The problem is the huge selection offered. So which do you choose? This depends solely on your preferences and needs. Some are looking for a snack; others use energy bars to replenish fuel after a long period of exercise. Some use energy bars as a meal replacement, and others simply like the taste and convenience. Remember "Energy" also means calories. Energy bars are another way to consume calories in a quick neat little package. Energy bars themselves will not provide magical powers to boost brainpower nor will they turn anyone into an Olympic athlete. The bottom line… they provide calories.

Whatever your reason for choosing an energy bar it is important to consider these factors:

- Check the label calories, these bars can range from 100- 400 calories.

- Choose a bar that is low in fat; less than 5 grams is reasonable.

- To replenish fuel during or after exercise look for bars with at least 25 grams of carbohydrates.

- Meal replacement bars should contain proportionately higher amounts of carbohydrates, protein, and fiber.

- Look at the sugar content; these can contain just as much sugar as a candy bar. Remember 1 tsp. of sugar is equal to 4 grams of sugar
- If you consume multiple bars a day you may be getting more vitamins and minerals than you need.
- Have some real food as a snack for variety; fruit is a great choice.
- Energy bars cannot be counted on to provide your daily fiber need. Isolated fibers, such as inulin, chicory, and oligosaccharides, may not provide the same benefit as fiber offered from food.

11 Popular Energy Bars

	Clif Kit's Organic Fruit Bar	Lara Bars	Picky Bars	Raw Revolution
Calories	190	200	150	200
Fat	12	12	5	7
Sat. Fat	1.5	3	6	1
Fiber	3	4	5	2
Protein	3	4	0	7
Carbs	22	25	24	28

	Healthy Warrior	Skout Bars	Clif Bars	Gatorade Bars	Kind Bars
Calories	100	190	240	260	190
Fat	5	7	4	5	12
Sat. Fat	1	1.5	1	1	1.5
Fiber	5	4	5	1	1
Protein	13	5	10	7	20
Carbs	13	30	41	47	15

	Luna Bars	ProBar Fruition
Calories	180	160
Fat	4	8
Sat. Fat	3	0.5
Fiber	2	3
Protein	10	6
Carbs	26	23

PIZZA: WHEN YOU KNEAD THE DOUGH

Pizza is a popular American food that is currently a $30 billion a year industry. Pizza can be a healthy addition to your diet if you make sensible selections. If not, two slices of pizza can add over 800 calories and a day's worth of sodium, cholesterol, and saturated fat to your intake. The popularity of pizza can add to the high incidence of heart disease in this country and our bulging waistlines.

A typical unhealthy pizza choice is Domino's Hand Tossed Pepperoni Pizza. One slice is equivalent to a McDonald's Egg McMuffin. Pizza Hut's Stuffed Crust Meat Lover's Pizza is equal to a McDonald's Big Mac, and who eats just one slice?

Frozen pizza plays a big part in the typical American's diet. It is currently the number one frozen dinner choice in this country. With the focus on improving food choices to reduce the incidence of obesity, many companies are beginning to offer more healthful pizza choices. Look at the charts following for some of these better choices for frozen pizza.

There are a number of healthy reasons to include pizza in your diet. Pizza sauce is rich in lycopene, an antioxidant that protects individuals against prostate and cervical cancers and reduces heart disease. It is also helps prevent eye disorders such as macular degeneration and cataracts that can lead to blindness. Pizza is a good source of lycopene due to its tomato sauce base. Cooked tomatoes contain 10 mg lycopene, which is more than fresh tomatoes. Vegetable pizzas, such as spinach, broccoli, and pepper can supply health benefits with their added contents of beta-carotene, folate, vitamin C, calcium, vitamin K, and anti-oxidants.

Cheese is a high source of calcium helpful in maintaining healthy teeth and bones. One slice of pizza can supply approximately 20% of the daily need for calcium. To reduce the fat and cholesterol content of pizza, look for part-skim mozzarella, which is leaner than traditional pizza cheeses. Many strict plant-based eaters choose soy cheese on their pizzas. Soy cheese has no cholesterol, lower saturated fat, and lower calories per slice. It is also helpful in lowering cholesterol levels in the body.

Pizza crust can be made with trans fats that increase heart disease risk. To insure a healthy crust, look for those made with whole wheat, oat bran, and wheat germ. Stay away from crusts with shortening and partially hydrogenated vegetable oil. Pizza can also supply over 30 percent of your recommended daily allowance for sodium in one slice. Excessive sodium intake can be a concern because it has been linked with high blood pressure and increased risk of stomach cancer. The adult recommended daily limit for sodium is 2300 mg. Compare pizza brands to ensure that a serving does not contain over 800 mg sodium. Make sure on days you choose pizza you limit your use of convenience foods, fast foods, and prepared foods that supply high amounts of sodium.

Suggestions for improving your pizza choices include:

- Order your pizza with half the cheese. Choose vegetable toppings that are lower in calories and higher in nutrition. Some companies add extra cheese with vegetable pizzas so make sure to check the calories. Chicken and ham are the next best choices. Try to avoid high-fat choices such as sausage, pork, and beef. Pepperoni is a better choice than these if the rest of your group is pushing meat pizzas. Another option would be to order half the pizza with meat and half without. This allows calorie and fat-hungry friends their choice and you get yours. If meat pizza is a favorite, having one slice with and one slice without will lower your calories, fat, and cholesterol intake.

FROZEN PIZZA

Pizza Brand	Calo-riesper Serving	Fat / Saturated Fat / Cholesterol	Carbs / Protein/ Sodium
A.C. LaRocco Tomato &Feta	251	7g Fat 2 g Saturated Fat 11 mg Cholesterol	39 g Carbohydrate 11 g Protein 341 mg Sodium
Amy's Pizza Cheese	305	12 g Fat 4 g Saturated Fat 15 mg Cholesterol	39 gr. Carbohydrate 12 g Protein 600 mg Sodium
Tombstone Original Pizza Extra Cheese	293	13 g Fat 6 g Saturated Fat 30 mg Cholesterol	32 g Carbohydrate 14 g Protein 586 mg Sodium
DiGiorno Rising Crust Spinach, Mushroom,and Garlic Pizza	262	8 g Fat 3 g Saturated Fat 17 mg Cholesterol	35 g Carbohydrate 12 g Protein 664 mg Sodium
Freshetta DiGiorno Brick OvenFire Baked Crust Roasted Portobello Mushrooms & Spinach	273	9 g Fat 4 g Saturated Fat 19 mg Cholesterol	36 g Carbohydrate 11 g Protein 602 mg Sodium

Wolfgang Puck Wood-Fired Thin Crust Vegetable	221	7 g Fat 3 g Saturated Fat 20 mg Cholesterol	29 g Carbohydrate 12 g Protein 449 mg Sodium
California Pizza Kitchen Barbequed Chicken	287	9 g Fat 5 g Saturated Fat 31 mg Cholesterol	34 g Carbohydrate 17 g Protein 717 mg Sodium
FreshettaSouthwest StyleChicken Supreme with Roasted RedPeppers	302	10 g Fat 4 g Saturated Fat 21 mg Cholesterol	40 g Carbohydrate 13 g Protein 965 mg Fat
Red Baron Pizzeria Style Special Deluxe	319	14 g Fat 5 g Saturated Fat 20 mg Cholesterol	36 g Carbohydrate 14 g Protein 824 mg Sodium

TAKE-OUT PIZZA

Sausage Pizza	Portion	Fat / Calories / Cholesterol	Carbs / Protein/ Sodium
Dominos - 12 inch	1/8	10 g / 191 / 28.5 mg	30 g / 7 g / 558 mg
Dominos - 14 inch	1/8	13 g / 267 / 28.5 mg	24 g / 12 g / 587 mg
Pizza Hut - 12 inch	1/8	18 g / 340 / 30 mg	— / 16 g / 910 mg
Papa Johns - 14 inch	1/8	18 g / 303 / 31 mg	24 g / 13 g / 724 mg
Vegetable Pizza			
Dominos - 12 inch	1/8	8 g / 220 / 17 mg	28 g / 9.5 g / 49 mg
Dominos - 14 inch	1/8	11 g / 302 / 38 mg	39 g / 13.2 g / 684 mg
Pizza Hut - 12 inch	1/8	8 g / 220 / 5 mg	29 g / 9 g / 580 mg
Papa Johns - 14 inch	1/8	11 g / 228 / 14 mg	24 g / 9 g / 447 mg

POPCORN: A PERFECTLY CRUNCHY SNACK

Popcorn is one of the most popular American snacks and 1.2 billion pounds of popcorn is consumed each year. Popcorn is high in whole grains, fiber, and polyphenol antioxidants. It contains 15 grams of fiber in 3.5-ounce servings and it is high in whole grains and polyphenol antioxidants This helps to reduce the risk of heart disease, diabetes, strokes, some cancers, and it improves gut health. It is also a rich source of protein, and iron. It has B complex vitamins and the minerals magnesium and manganese.

Popcorn can be an unhealthy snack depending on how much you eat, what you put on it, and the type you are eating. Since it is easy to overeat when consuming popcorn, be sure to check out the serving sizes when you sit down to eat .

1. Read the label and look for sugar and sodium contents. A healthy snack should range between 100-150 calories. It should also have less than 5 grams sugar and 150 milligrams of sodium.

2. Check for saturated fat contents that should be between 5-10 percent of your daily calories. Many microwave and movie popcorns have 25 percent of daily saturated fat that could be harmful to your heart.

3. Check the serving size of each popcorn you have selected. Then check the number of servings the popcorn contains. Measure your portion into a bowl.

Check out the portion differences between popcorns. Notice that the biggest issue with movie popcorn is the amount provided in each regular, large, and super-size selection. The Dollar store, Michaels, and Amazon sell plastic popcorn containers that allow for approximately 3- 3 1/2 cups of popcorn. Throw in your purse and measure movie popcorn into this container. This shows what 3 ½ cups looks like. For an occasional treat, a 3 ½ cup serving is okay, but 11-24 cups is excessive and contains almost a whole day's calories, sodium, fat, and saturated fat.

Types	Regular (no butter) (3 serv.) MOVIE	Regular (no butter) (1 serv.)	Large (6 serv.) MOVIE	Large (1 serv.) MOVIE	Super-Size (8 serv.) MOVIE	Super-size (1 serv.) MOVIE	Air-Popped Butter	Skinny pop	Orville Redenbacher Classic Butter	Pop Secret Butter Popcorn	Skinny Girl Butter Salt Popcorn
Servings (cups)	11 cups	3 ½ cups	20 cups	3 ½ cups	24 cups	3 ½ cups	3 cups	3 ¾ cups	3 ½ cups	3 ½ cups	3 cups
Calories	700	200	1330	371	1680	480	100	150	170	160	80
Fat (grams)	27	7	51	15	64	15	1	10	12	10	3
Saturated Fat (grams)	34	10	60	17	67	19	0	1	6	5	1

Diacetyl, that serves as a buttery flavoring in microwave popcorn, has been questioned as a possible toxic product. Many workers in popcorn factories have developed lung disease from breathing in the chemical. Many companies have eliminated its use, adding another chemical with a similar chemical form that appears to be as harmful. Continued research needs to be done to ensure that people eating normal amounts of popcorn are not at risk.

The product, perflurooctanoic acid (PFOA) is used in the linings of microwave bags , pizza boxes, and Teflon. There has been considerable concern about its use due to the fact that (PFOA) is found in the blood of almost all Americans. PFOA can be removed by the body or it can stay in the body for years. Increased cancer has been found in animals, but the relationship is not as clear in humans. Research continues on its safety.

SUSHI: DANCING TO
A DIFFERENT TUNA

Sushi is a popular Japanese food that has become very popular in the United States. It can be found in grocery stores, restaurants, and bars. It is also a food that can be eaten on the run. Sushi can be cold, cooked, or topped with sweet vinegar. It is often filled with raw, cooked, or marinated fish. Shellfish, eggs, or vegetables can also be used for fillers.

Sushi can be made in a variety of ways including hand-formed, rolled, or pressed. It can be made into small bite-sized pieces or large rolls. It is often made with sliced raw fish called sashimi.

Sushi is a nutritious food that is low in calories, low in sodium when limited condiments are used, and low fat unless fried or very fatty fish are used. It is an excellent source of carbohydrate, protein, and other nutrients depending on the types used. Check the lists below for your best choices and those items you should look out for.

GOOD SUSHI CHOICES:

- Try sushi served steamed, grilled, or boiled.
- Use low sodium soy sauce or Tamari sauce or limit use of added condiments to minimize sodium intake

Chose reputable restaurants, grocery stores, or bars to ensure that the raw fish you are eating is fresh. A few tips for ensuring the safety of fish is to go to places that have a large customer base. This will increase the chances that the fish served or sold is being turned over fast. Take a look in the kitchen on the way to the restroom. Does it look clean and neat? Fresh sushi should have a clean water smell. If the fish you are being served has a fishy smell, it is probably not fresh and should be avoided.

- Order steamed veggies like hijiki (cooked sea weed) or Ooshi-tashi (boiled spinach) with soy sauce to fill up.

- Pick soups and sashimi that tend to be lower in calories. Consider sukiyaki that is meat or vegetables usually served at the table in a shallow pan or Teppanyaki dishes that are meat, fish, or vegetables cooked on an iron griddle.

- Order brown rice in place of white rice because it retains many nutrients that are lost in processing white rice. These include: iron, vitamin B, vitamin B3, and Magnesium. Brown rice wrapped in nori (dried seaweed) has iodine, zinc, cilium, vitamins A, E, C, and K. It is also higher in fiber and protein.

- Wasabi sauce (hot green paste) is a Japanese horseradish that is served with sashimi. It can help you from having food poisoning due to its antimicrobial properties.

- Ginger is served with sushi in a pickled form to cleanse the palate after each sushi piece. Ginger contains the compounds gingerols and shogaols that stimulate digestive juices and neutralize stomach acids. It is effective in blocking the body's vomit reflex. It also helps lower cholesterol and limits blood clotting like aspirin.

- Mackerel is a great sushi choice due to its omega-3 fatty acids, low mercury levels, and selenium levels that work along with the omegas to neutralize free radicals.

- Drink green tea as your beverage to help lower total cholesterol and improve the ratio of HDL (good cholesterol) to LDL (bad cholesterol). It is also a zero-calorie choice.

WATCH OUT FOR:

- Be careful with tempura vegetables or seafood that are cooked in batter and deep-fried. This choice can add extra calories, fat, and cholesterol depending on the type of oil used.
- Stay clear of teriyaki or yaketori sauce that both have a considerable amount of sugar that can add calories.
- Sake can add a considerable number of calories having 40-calories/ounce.
- Avoid spicy items that tend to be higher in calories and fat due to the sauces that usually have added mayonnaise.
- Restrict use of red bluefish tuna due to its high mercury content and (PCB's), organic compounds that can cause harm to the brain and endocrine system.
- Avoid tobiko sushi that is made of fish roe and quail eggs due to the high cholesterol and saturated fat content. Since they are eaten raw, there is a risk of salmonella poisoning.

The FDA has recommended that individuals who are pregnant or those with compromised immune systems should avoid the use of raw fish. These would include children, elderly, and those with liver disease, diabetes, and other autoimmune disorders. This is due to the higher risk of severe outcomes from infection from spoiled raw fish.

Sushi	Serving	Carbs	Protein (g)	Sodium Size (g)	Calories (g)	Fat (g)
California Roll	4 pieces	150	25	4	4	170
Dragon Roll	4 pieces	290	28	10	3	300
Shrimp Nigiri	4 pieces	130	18	12	1	620
Shrimp Tempura Roll	6 pieces	220	12	10	13	500
Cooked Soybeans	1/2 cup	100	9	8	3	310
Spicy Salmon Roll	6 pieces	160	16	8	7	560
Spicy Tuna Roll	6 pieces	100	16	8	7	430
Spider Roll (soft shell crab)	3 pieces	200	20	11	9	620
Summer Roll	1 roll	130	14	10	9	90
Vegetable Roll	5 pieces	120	22	3	3	520

CARNIVAL, MOVIE, AND STADIUM FARE

Carnival, fair, and stadium foods can be particularly high in calories and poor in nutrition. Check out the calories and nutrition information listed. If you look forward to a particular food at a favorite event, try the following:

- Eat smaller meals leading up to the snack.
- Use your extra calories to put towards your particular favorite snack
- Eat a meal before you go. When going to a ball game, we have a tradition to eat a lunch or dinner before to handle calories more easily and to get foods that are more to our taste.
- You can always share a snack with a friend. Portions served are generally large.

Know what you will experience with foods before you go. Have fun and do your best to keep calorie goals and food strategies in mind.

Food	Carbs (g)	Protein (g)	Fat (g)	Calories (Kcal)
1/3 lb. Hot Dog	31	14	41	550
Foot Long Hot Dog	41	18	26	470
Corndog, 4 oz	36	8	21	250
French Fries, 7 oz	70	16	24	560
Cheese Fries, 10 oz	62	14	38	645
Onion Rings, 3 rings	40	8	13	310
Cole Slaw, 5 oz	37	3	21	350
Kettle Corn, 5 oz	110	6	15	600
Kettle Corn, 10 oz	220	12	30	1200
Funnel Cake, plain	80	11	44	760
Funnel Cake, cinnamon/sugar	88.5	11	44	790
Strawberries & Cream	96		8	830
Churro, 1 oz	21	9	8	165
Cotton Candy, 5.5 oz	156			625
Soft Pretzel, 4.5 oz	70	10.5	2	240
Soft Pretzel, 8 oz	147	20.7	5	710
Candied Apple, 7 oz	80		0.5	330
Snow Cone, 3 oz	68			270
Slushie, 16 oz	65			260
Malt, 16 oz	85		33	690

It is better to think of creative and lower calorie ways to enjoy your favorite snacks than to overeat and feel bad. Cutting out favorite snacks completely may cause upset that will result in later sabotage of your newly formed food behaviors.

CONCLUSION

So, here you are at the end of *Too Busy to Diet*. Perhaps you were just looking for some healthy menu ideas to add variety to your meals, or maybe you wanted to learn more about adding fiber or calcium to your diet. We hope *Too Busy to Diet* has served as a road map, helping you navigate the maze of eating situations that you face daily.

We've covered the nutrition topics that we think reflect the health concerns you might have. We believe the "Fab Five," weight, cholesterol, fiber, calcium, and exercise, are essential chapters for being healthy. Make sure to re-read them when you have a moment.

We know over the years you've been bombarded with nutrition information: TV and radio shows, web sites, magazines, books, and "wannabe nutritionists." In fact, there probably isn't a woman's magazine out there that doesn't supply us with nutrition information on a regular basis. Some is good information, some is not so good. Look for articles written by registered dietitians. Today, magazines use registered dietitians as the "Nutrition Experts."

We hope we've provided the right information in just the right amount, enabling you to make the right choices. By now you may be shopping, reading food labels, and sitting down more often to a home cooked meal. Maybe you've even tried some delicious recipes that take less time to fix than stopping at a restaurant or waiting for carry out food. We hope so.

We think you'll find *Too Busy to Diet* is a great traveling companion or bedside reference. Our fundamental goal was to provide you with a guide that makes healthy living easy. We wish you healthy and happy eating.

Jackie & Monica

SECTION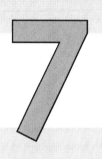

APPENDIX

APPENDIX A: SAMPLE MEAL PLANS FOR WEIGHT LOSS AND WEIGHT MAINTENANCE

This table shows sample meal plans that show the number of servings for different caloric levels. If you are at your healthy weight, choose a caloric level that is close to what you are currently eating. If you need to lose or gain weight, a registered dietitian can help you determine your caloric and specific nutritional needs.

Calories Daily	1200	1400	1600	1800	2000	2200
Carbohydrate / Starch (15 g carb/ serving)	6	6	8	8	9	10
Vegetables (5 g carb/serving)	3	3	3	3	3	3
Fruit (15 g carb/servings)	3	4	4	5	6	6
Milk & Yogurt (12 g carb/serving)	2	2	3	3	3	4
Protein 7 g protein/ serving	5	6	6	6	7	8
Fat (5 g fat /serving)	1	3	3	5	6	6

APPENDIX B: MONTH OF MEALS

BREAKFAST MEAL PLANS

Meal plans were developed showing the food components that should be included daily for good nutrition. The below symbols represent these food components. Please note that some of the meals may be missing some of the food components. This accounts for days when you are in a rush or are saving your food for a holiday meal or a larger meal out. It is encouraged that you attempt to eat all of the food components at each meal when you can. Make up for missed foods at snacks or save for a larger meal later in the day when needed.

Chart Key	
F	High Fiber
H	Heart Healthy
C	Calcium Rich

* pick healthy margarine choices when possible

1 small whole wheat bagel F H	2 low-fat, whole wheat waffles F H
1 slice 2% cheese slice	1 tbs. lite syrup
C H 1/3 cantaloupe	2 tsp. soft tub margarine H
F H 1 cup skim milk H C	1 ¼ cups fresh strawberries F H
1 cup blueberries F H	1 cup skim milk H C

1 cup 80-100 calorie low-fat yogurt C H ¼ cup low fat granola F H 1 slice whole wheat toast F H 1 tsp. soft tub margarine H Small fresh orange F H	1 ½ cups Cheerios F H 1 slice whole wheat toast F H 1 tsp. soft tub margarine H Small banana F H 1 cup skim milk H C
1 cup cooked oatmeal F H 2 tbs. raisins F H 1 cup skim milk H C	Large whole wheat bagel F H 1 tbs. lite cream cheese H 1 cup skim milk or 100-calorie yogurt H C
1 slice leftover thin cheese pizza C Small fresh apple F H	Granola bar F H 1 cup 100-calorie yogurt F H 17 grapes F H

¼ cup low-fat cottage cheese C H 1 unsweetened pineapple half F H 2 slices raisin toast F H 2 tsp. soft tub margarine H	Whole wheat English muffin F H 1 tbs. peanut butter H Small fresh peach F H 1 cup skim milk H C
Cupcake-size low-fat bran muffin F H 1 tsp. soft tub margarine H 1 cup 100-calorie, low-fat yogurt H C Small fresh pear F H	2 slices whole wheat toast F H scrambled egg with 1 slice 2% fat cheese C 1 tsp. soft tub margarine H Half grapefruit F H
2 slices French whole wheat toast F H 2 tsp. soft tub margarine H 1 tbs. lite syrup 1 cup 100-calorie, low-fat yogurt H C small fresh banana F H	2 medium whole wheat pancakes F H 1 tbs. lite syrup 1 cup blueberries F H 1 cup skim milk H C

Cheese omelet (made with 1 egg white and 2 egg whites):

2% fat cheese (1 slice) C

1 egg and 2 egg whites

slices whole wheat toast F H

1 orange F H

Whole wheat English muffin F H

1 slice 2% fat cheese C H

1 fresh apple F H

3 graham cracker squares F H

2 tbsp. peanut butter H

1 cup skim milk H C
Tangerine F H

Breakfast burrito: 1 scrambled egg

1 whole wheat tortilla F H 1 slice

2% fat cheese H C Salsa

Fresh fruit cup F H

1 hard-boiled egg

Granola bar F H 100-calorie,

low-fat yogurt H C Small banana F H

whole wheat English muffin F H

1-ounce slice lean ham H

light pineapple rings F H

1 cup skim milk H C

Thomas 100-cal whole wheat English muffin F H

2 tsp. soft tub margarine H

1 cup 100-calorie, low-fat yogurt H
C 1 small banana F H

Thomas 100-cal whole wheat bagel
F H 2 tsp. soft tub margarine H

1 cup 100-calorie low-fat yogurt HC

1 small pear FH

½ cup trail mix F H

1 cup 100-calorie, low-fat yogurt H C

1 cup 100-calorie, low-fat yogurt H C

¼ cup grape nuts F H

1 small banana F H

Peanut butter and Jelly toast:
1 tbsp. peanut butter H

tsp. all-fruit jelly

2 slices whole wheat toast F H
1 cup skim milk H C

1 ¼ c. Strawberries F H

1 whole wheat pita F H

¼ cup low-fat cottage cheese H C

1 small banana sliced F H

Granola F H Yogurt H C Mixed berries F H	Fresh fruit kabob (can include: strawberries, grapes, blueberries, and other fresh fruits of your liking) F H 1 Cranberry Orange low-fat muffin F H/Skim milk H C
Lox with cucumbers, sliced tomatoes, on mixed greens F H Small whole wheat bagel F H Low-fat cream cheese H Fresh Grapes and Strawberries F H Skim milk H C	Breakfast Quesadilla: Whole wheat tortilla F H Fresh Fruit cup F H 1 slice 2% fat cheddar cheese C H

LUNCH MEAL PLANS

Vegetarian Choices are marked in parenthesis to allow the entire family to eat the same base meal with the vegetarian alternate provided for the vegetarian member.

Chart Key	
F	High Fiber
H	Heart Healthy
C	Calcium Rich

* pick healthy margarine choices when possible

2-4 ounces grilled salmon H Mixed greens F H (Hard cooked egg and cheese slices or feta cheese C) 2 tbs. lite salad dressing H Large whole wheat roll F H Large apple F H	2 small soft whole wheat tortillas F H 2-4 ounces grilled chicken (black beans) F H ((1 ounce grated 2 % cheese) C H) Lettuce/tomato F H Large orange F H

2 slices whole wheat bread F H
2-4 ounces turkey H
((scrambled eggs)
Lettuce/tomato F H)
Large pear F H

1 cup vegetable soup F H
6 whole wheat crackers F H
(2 slices 2% fat cheese C)
34 grapes F H

1 cup homemade chili made with lean beef or turkey F H
(vegetarian chili) F H
1-ounce grated cheese C
Apple F H
Vegetable omelet F
2 slices whole wheat toast F H
2 tsp. lite margarine H
Fresh fruit cup F H

60-90 calorie yogurt H C
Fresh apple F H
2 tbs. peanut butter H
Small low-fat muffin H
1 tsp. lite margarine H

2-4 ounces water-packed tuna H
((2 slices 2 % cheese) C)
2 slices whole wheat bread F H
1 tsp. lite mayonnaise H
Lettuce/tomatoes, Raw carrots F H
Large peach F H

2 slices whole wheat bread F H
(2 tbs. peanut butter H)
1 tsp. no-sugar jelly
1 ¼ cups strawberry F H

Frozen luncheon meal (frozen veg-etarian meal)
Salad F H/2 tbs. lite salad dressing H
Slice of whole wheat bread F H
2 small tangerines F H

1 cup chicken noodle soup
6 whole wheat crackers F H
(2 slice 2% fat cheese) C H
Small plum F H

2-4 ounces grilled chicken H
(hard cooked egg and 2 oz 2% cheese)
Mixed greens F H
2 tbs. lite salad dressing H
2 large bread sticks
1 cup diet applesauce F H

2-4 ounces grilled fish
(2/3 cup brown rice) F H
(2/3 cup kidney beans) F H
Steamed broccoli F H C
Salad F H
2 tbs. lite salad dressing H
Fresh pear F H
Low calorie lunch:
50 calorie high fiber tortilla F H
((2) 50 calorie 2% cheese
2 slices or turkey) slices C H
Large fresh fruit F H

Low calorie lunch:
100 calorie whole wheat English
muffin F H
2 slices 50 calorie cheese C H
Large fresh fruit F H

Lunch on the run:
Slim fast or Carnation Instant
Breakfast C
Fresh Fruit F H
1 starch (pretzels, roll, crackers)

Leftover manicotti, lasagna C (VEG)
Salad F H
2 tbs. lite dressing H
Fresh orange F H

Trail Mix F H
(300 calorie portion)
100 calorie, low-fat yogurt H C

---

2 ounces peanut butter pretzels H
Fresh fruit F H

100 calorie, low-fat yogurt H C
Fresh fruit F H
Whole wheat roll F H

---

2 Mozzarella sticks H C
Fresh fruit F H
Whole wheat Crackers F H

Energy bar with at least 10 g protein
Fresh fruit F H

Macaroni and cheese C
Salad F H
2 tbs. lite dressing H
Fresh Peach F H

Egg salad
Hard-cooked eggs
Low fat mayonnaise H
Celery F H
High fiber tortilla F H
Fresh pear F H

Hummus F H

Lettuce and Tomato F H

Whole wheat tortilla F H

Fresh grapes F H

Chicken salad (peanut butter sandwich)

Chopped chicken H

Low-fat mayonnaise H

Celery F H

Whole wheat toast F H

Fresh plums F H

Chicken Strips H (beans and rice)

Mixed Baby Greens F H

Oil and vinegar H

Whole wheat roll F H

Margarine H

Fresh orange F H

Roasted turkey roll H (egg salad)

2 (cheese slices)

Low fat Coleslaw F

Spinach tortilla F H

Fresh orange F H

DINNER MEAL PLANS

Vegetarian Choices are marked in parenthesis to allow the entire family to eat the same base meal with the vegetarian alternate provided for the vegetarian member.

Chart Key

F	High Fiber
H	Heart Healthy
C	Calcium Rich

* pick healthy margarine choices when possible

Frozen dinner meal

(vegetarian frozen meal)

Salad with tomatoes, raw vegetables

F H

1 tsp. olive oil and vinegar H

Small whole wheat roll F H

1 ¼ cup fresh strawberries F H

Grilled chicken breast H

(2/3 cup kidney, black, or garbanzo beans) F H

(2/3 cup brown rice) F H

½ cup green beans F H

(fresh salad) F H

2 tbs. lite salad dressing H

Fresh apple F H

Baked orange roughy H

(2 % fat grated cheese) H C

Large baked potato with skin F H

2 tbs. lite sour cream H

Broccoli F H C

Fresh orange F H

Lamb chop H

(chicken textured protein) H

(grilled Portobello mushroom) F H

1 cup whip potatoes

½ cup carrots F H

Salad F H

2 tbs. lite salad dressing H

Fresh watermelon F H

Pork tenderloin H

(tofu) H

Stir-fry vegetables F H

1 cup whole wheat pasta F H

fresh salad F H

2 tbs. lite salad dressing H

Fresh blueberries (1 cup) F H

(½ cup of hummus H F)

2 small spinach tortillas F H

Tomato F H

Lettuce F H

Salad F H

2 tbs. lite salad dressing H

½ cup mandarin oranges F H

Lean hamburger H (veggie burger) H Hamburger bun Lettuce/tomato F H

½ cup mushrooms F H

Fresh grapes F H

Vegetable omelet

2 slices whole wheat toast F H

2 tsp. lite margarine H

Fresh cantaloupe F H

---

2 slices whole wheat toast F H

2-4 ounces tuna H

(2 slices 2 % cheese slices) C H

Lite mayonnaise H

Raw celery sticks F H

Fresh peach F H

½ cups whole wheat pasta F H

Lean meat sauce (tomato sauce) H

2 tbs. parmesan cheese C

Large mixed salad F H

2 tbs. lite salad dressing H

Large banana F H

2 small soft whole wheat tortillas F H

2-3 oz grilled chicken, lean turkey, or beef H

(2/3 cup kidney, garbanzo, or black beans) H F

1 ounce 2% fat grated cheese C H
Lettuce/ tomatoes F H

Large Apple F H

2 slices thin sliced cheese or vegetable pizza C

Fresh salad F H

2 tbs. lite salad dressing H

½ cup fruit cup F H

Pork chop H (tofu) H

2/3 cup brown rice F H

Pineapple slices/green peppers F H
Salad F H

2 tbs. lite salad dressing H

Chicken roll-up with 3 ounces chicken slices H

(kidney, garbanzo, or black beans) H F
1 ounce grated 2% fat cheese C H
Lettuce F H

Light mayonnaise
Salad F H

1 tsp. olive oil and vinegar H

½ mango F H

Large baked potato with skin F H
2-4 ounces 2% fat cheese C H
Broccoli F H C

2 tbs. lite sour cream H
Salad F H

2 tbs. lite salad dressing H
Large fresh pear F H

Grilled cheese sandwich: (made with 2% fat cheese, lite margarine, 2 slices whole wheat bread) C F H

1 cup vegetable soup F H

½ cup natural applesauce F H

4 ounces steak (veggie burger)

½ cup green beans F H

Baked potato with skin F H
1 tbs. lite sour cream H
Salad F H

2 tbs. lite salad dressing H
Fresh small banana F H

Grilled tuna sandwich on a whole wheat bun or whole wheat English muffin F H

(grilled eggplant) F H

(1-ounce mozzarella cheese) C H
Raw carrots and celery F H
Large fresh Apple F H

1 cup whole wheat spaghetti F H Chicken strips H (marinara sauce) Salad F H 1 tsp. olive oil and vinegar H Small peach F H	4 ounces grilled salmon H (kidney, garbanzo, or black beans) H F (tempeh or Seitan) Broccoli F H C 1 cup brown rice F H Salad F H tbs. lite salad dressing H 2 small plums F H
1 cup meat chili F H (1 c. vegetarian chili with beans) F H 1 ounce 2% fat cheese C H Salad F H tbs. lite salad dressing H Small orange F H	Pork stir-fry H (tofu or vegetable stir-fry) F H Sugar snap peas F H cup brown rice F H Salad F H tbs. lite salad dressing H 1 cup blueberries F H
½ cup chili beans F H 1 ounce 2% fat grated cheese C 2 small whole wheat tortillas F H Salad F H 1 banana	4 ounces Tilapia H (lentils) F H 1 cup couscous F H Broccoli HCF/Salad FH 2 tbs. lite salad dressing H 1/3 cantaloupe F H
Frozen cheese ravioli C Tomato sauce Salad F H 2 tbs. lite salad dressing H 1 ¼ cup strawberries F H	Roast turkey H (butternut or spaghetti squash) F H 1 cup stuffing Salad F H 1 tsp. olive oil and vinegar H Small peach F H

Round steak H

(veggie sausage or soyrizo) H

Green peppers F H

1 cup brown rice F H

Salad F H

2 tbs. salad dressing H

1 cup watermelon F H

Hearty bean soup F H

French bread

Salad F H

2 tbs. lite salad dressing H

1 cup fruit salad F H

Gnocchi

Meat sauce (marina sauce)

Salad F H

2 tbs. lite dressing H

1 cup berries F H

½ cup no fat Cottage cheese H C

Whole wheat roll F H

1 tsp. lite margarine H

1 cup fruit cocktail F H

Macaroni and cheese C

Fresh salad F H

2 tbs. lite dressing H

Small apple F H

Roasted turkey roll H (Tempeh)

(vegetarian dinner)

Low fat Coleslaw H F

Spinach tortilla F H

Fresh orange F H

Vegetable lasagna C F

Salad F H

2 tbs. lite dressing H

Small apple F H

Cheese quesadillas C

Lettuce and tomato F H

Vegetable soup F H

1/3 cantaloupe F H

Peanut butter sandwich on whole

wheat bread F H

Raw celery sticks F H

1/3 honeydew melon F H

APPENDIX C:
SUGGESTED RESOURCES

1. Price, Jessie. The Simple Art of Eating Well Test Kitchen.

2. Hornick, Betsy & Chamberlain, Richard. The Healthy Beef Cookbook National Cattlemen's Beef Association. John Wiley & Sons, 2006

3. Napier, Kristine & Food and Culinary Professionals

   American Dietetic Association Cooking. Healthy Across America. American Dietetic Association. John Wiley & Sons, 2004

4. Duyff, Roberta Larson, MS, RD, FADA, CFS. 365 Days of Healthy Eating from the American Dietetic Association. John Wiley & Sons, 2003

5. Castle, Stacie, RD; Cotler, Robyn, RD; Scheftner, Marni, RD; Shapiro, Shana, RD. Bite it & Write It: A Guide to Keeping Track of What You Eat & Drink. Square One Publishing, 2011

6. Lindberg, Alexander, MD. Eating the Greek Way. Clarkson Potter Publications, 2007

7. Ponichtera, Brenda J.,RD. Quick and Healthy Recipes and Ideas. Small Steps Press,2008

8. Ponichtera, Brenda J., RD. Quick and Healthy Volume II Small Steps Press, 2009

9. Nelson, Miriam E., PhD. Strong Women Stay Young. Bantam Book, 2005

10. Rondinielli, Lara, RD, CDE & Bucko, Jennifer Healthy Eating Calendar Diabetic Cooking. American Diabetes Association, 2004

11. Borushek, Allan. Calorie King Calorie, Fat, and Carbohydrate Counter. 2012 www.calorieking.com

12. Davis, Brenda, RD & Melinda, Vesanto, MS, RD with Berry, Ryan. Becoming Raw: The Essential Guide to Raw Vegan Diets

13. Adle, Karen & Fertig, Judith. The Gardner & the Grill: The Bounty of the Garden Meets the Sizzle of the Grill

SUGGESTED APPLICATIONS

1. CalorieCount.com

2. LoseIt.com

3. WebMD.com Food and Fitness Planner

4. MyFitnessPal.com

5. SparkPeople.com

6. EatingWell.com/menuplanner

7. MealSnap.com

8. Whole Foods Market app

9. AllRecipes.com Dinner Spinner

10. Kelloggsnutrition.com/fiber-tracker-mobile/

11. Calorieking.com

12. RealSimple.com

SUGGESTED MAGAZINES

1. www.CleanEating.com
2. www.EatingWell.com
3. www.CookingLight.com
4. Food & Nutrition, Academy of Nutrition and Dietetics

APPENDIX D:
REFERENCES

References

1. Alexandria D Blatt, Roe, L.S. Barbara & Rolls, J. (2011) Hidden vegetables: An Effective Strategy to Reduce Energy Intake and Increase Vegetable Intake in Adults, American Journal of Clinical Nutrition, February 2011,

2. American Dietetic Association Position Statement on Superfoods. Neuhouser ML, Wassertheil-Smoller S, Thomson C et al. (2009).

3. "Multivitamin Use and Risk of Cancer and Cardiovascular Disease in the Women's Health Initiative Cohorts"; July 31, 2018, Journal of American college of Cardiology

4. *Arch Internal Medicine, vol.169 No.3, February 9, 2009.* Andrew Freeman, MD., Director, Cardiovascular Prevention and Wellness, National Jewish Health, Denver; Angela Lemond, RDN, LD., Spokesperson, Academy of Nutrition and Dietetics; July 31, 2018,

5. HealthDay July 23, 2018 JAMA, 2019:321 (11) : 1081-1093, Victor N. Zhang PhD et al.

6. Zhang, Victor N., PhD et al, Association of Dietary Cholesterol or Egg Consumption with Incident of Cardiovascular Disease and Mortality, JAMA, 2019:321 (11) : 1081-1093.

7. American Heart Association. "Coffee May Help Perk Up your Blood Vessels."ScienceDaily, 20 November 2013.

8. American Heart Association (AHA), Statement On Caffeine. (2007). http://www. Americanheart.org/presenter.jhtml

9. American Heart Association. Carbohydrates and Sugars. Accessed April 20, 2010. http://www.Americanheart.org/ presenter

10. Diet Quality Indexes and Mortality in Postmenopausal Women: The Iowa Women's Health Study. Jaakko Mursu, Lyn M Steffen, Katie A Meyer, Daniel Duprez, David R Jacobs, Jr.

11. *The American Journal of Clinical Nutrition*, Volume 98, Issue 2, August 2013, Pages 444–453, https://doi.org/10.3945/ ajcn.112.055681

12. Andersen, L.F., Jacobs, D.R, Jr, Carlsen, M.H., Blomhoff, Rune. Consumption of Coffee is Associated with Reduced Risk of Death Attributed to Inflammatory and Cardiovascular Diseases in the Iowa Women's Health Study. *Am. J. Clinical Nutrition*, May 2006; 83: 1039

13. Bischoff-Ferrari HA, Willett WC, Wong JB, Giovannucci E, Dietrich T, Dawson- Hughes B. Fracture Prevention with Vitamin D Supplementation: A Meta-analysis of Randomized Controlled Trials. *JAMA*. 2005; 293:2257

14. Boonen S, Lips P, Bouillon R, Bischoff-Ferrari HA, Vanderschueren D, Haentjens, Need for Additional Calcium to Reduce the Risk of Hip Fractures with Vitamin D Supplementation: Evidence from a Comparative Meta-analysis of Randomized Controlled Trials. *J Clin Endocrinol Metab*. 2007; 92:1415-23.

15. Brenner, MD, Northwestern University, Feinberg School of Medicine, Chicago, Il. "Probiotics for the Treatment of Adult Gastrointestinal Disorders", July 2011.

16. Cnattingius, S., Signorello, L.B., Anneren, G., Clausson, B., Ekbom, A., Ljunger, E., Blot, W.J., McLaughlin, J.K., Petersson, G., Rane, A., Granath, F. Caffeine Intake and the Risk of First-trimester Spontaneous Abortion. *N Eng J Med.* 2000; Dec 21; 343(25):1839-1845.

17. Coffee, Tea, and Fatal Oral/Pharyngeal Cancer in a Large Prospective U.S. Cohort. Published online December 9, 2012 in the *American Journal of Epidemiology*. First author Janet S. Hildebrand, MPH, American Cancer Society, Atlanta, Ga.

18. Community Gardening; Wikipedia, en.wikipedia.orgwiki/Community_gardening

19. Economic Costs of Diabetes in the U.S. in 2007., Diabetes Care, March 2008, vol 31,no.3, 596-615

20. Dietary Reference Intakes: Food and Nutrition Board of Institute of Medicine National Academy Press, Wash. D.C., 7/29/2011

21. Dr. Kevin D. Hall PhD, Sachs, G. PhD, Chandramohen, D. BSc, Chow, CC, PhD, Y. Claire Wang, Y.C. MD, Steven L. Gortmaker PhD, Boyd A. Swinburn MD. Quantification of the Effect of Energy Imbalance On Bodyweight. The Lancet Volume 378, Issue 9793, pages 826-837, 2011, August 27.

22. E. Ekblom-Bak, B., Ekblom, Vikstrom, M.Hellenius, ML British Journal of Sports Medicine 2013. The Importance of Non-exercise Physical Activity for Cardiovascular Health and Longetivity

23. EFSA (2015). Scientific Opinion On The Safety of Caffeine, ESFA Journal,13(5):4102.

24. Martinez-Lapiscina, Elena, H et.al. Journal of Neurology, Neurosurgery and Psychiatry, 2013; 84 (12); 13-1325

25. Environmental Working Group. Sugar in Children's Cereals, http://ww.ewg.org/ report/sugar-in-children's-Cereals/more_sugar-25

26. Essential Guide to Vitamins and Minerals: Second Edition, Revised and Updated by Elizabeth Somer, Health Media of America, 1/14, 96. Harper Collins Publishers, 10 East 53rd St., New York, New York 10022

27. Food & Nutrition, November/December 2013, Academy of Nutrition and Dietetics, Sweet Stuff, Kerry Neville, pg. 16-17.

28. Food and Nutrition Magazine, March 15, *2019 Menopause* and Weight *Gain, Diana* Reid

29. Martin, Francois-Pierre, Rezzi, J, Serge, Per-Trepat, E., Kamlage, B., Collino, S. ,Leibold, E., Kastler, J., Rein, D., Fay, L. B., and Kochhar, SI. Metabolic Effects of Dark Chocolate Consumption on Energy, Gut Microbiota, and Stress-Related Metabolism in Free-Living Subjects, *Journal of Proteome Research*, 2009.

30. Freeman, MD., Director, Andrew, Cardiovascular Prevention and Wellness, National Jewish Health, Denver; Angela, Leman R.D.N., LD., Spokesperson, Academy of Nutrition and Dietetics; July 31, 2018, Journal of American College of Cardiology, online.

31. Good, CK. Holschuh NM, Albertson A.M., Eldridge A.L. Whole Grain Consumption and Body Mass Index in Adult Women: An Analysis of NHANES 1999-2000 and the USDA Pyramid Serving Database. J Am Cull Nutr 2008; 27:80-7.

32. Gorin AA, Phelan S., Hill JO, and Wing RR. (2004). Medical Triggers are Associated with Better Short-and Long-term Weight Loss Outcomes. *Preventive Medicine*, 39, 612-16.

33. Gorin AA, Phelan S, Wing R.R., Hill JO. (2004). Promoting Long Term Weight Control: Does Dieting Consistency Matter? *International Journal of Obesity and Related Metabolic Disorders*, 28, 278-8 Brinkworth, Gavin D., PhD.

34. Buckley, J.D, PhD; Noakes, M, PhD; Clifton, PhD; Wilson, C.D., PhD. Long-term Effects of a Very Low-Carbohydrate Diet and a Low-Fat Diet on Mood and Cognitive Function, *Arch Intern Med.* 2009; 169(20): 1873-1880.

35. Hamnid R., Farshchi, T. Moira J., and Mac Donald., I., Increased LDl. Levels Deleterious Effects of Omitting Breakfast on Insulin Fasting Lipids, American Journal of Clinical Nutrition, February 2005 vol 81(2)388-396.

36. Health.com. Can Pedialyte Really Help a Hangover? January 29, 2019.

37. Holick MF. Vitamin D Deficiency. *N Engl J Med.* 2007; 357:266-81Holick MF. Vitamin D: Importance in the Prevention of Cancers, Type 1 Diabetes, Heart disease, and Osteoporosis. *Am J Clin Nutr.* 2004; 79:362-71.

38. Holt, S.H., Miller, J.C., Petocz, D, Farmakalidis, E. Department of Biochemistry University of Sydney, Australia: A Satiety Index of Common Foods, European Journal of Clinical Nutrition, 1995 Sept; 49 (9): 675-90.

39. I-min, Lee, Djousse, L., et.al, JAMA, 2010; 303(12) 1173-1179. Physical Activity and Weight Gain Prevention.

40. Institute of Medicine. *Dietary Reference Intakes for Calcium and Vitamin D.* Washington, D.C.: National Academies Press, 2010.

41. Shal, Iris, RD, Ph.D, Schwarzfuch, M.D., D. Henkin, Y., M.D. Sshahar, D., R..D., Ph.D., Witkow, S., R.D., M.P.H., Greenberg, L., R.D., M.P.H., Golan, R., lR.D., M.P.H., Fraser, D., Ph.D., Bolotin, A., Ph.D, Hilel V., M.Sc., Tangi-Rozental, O., B.A. Zuk-Ramot, R., R.N., Sarusi, B., M.Sc., Brickner, D., M.D., Fiedler, M.D. ,Z, Bluher, M.,M.D. Stumvoll, M.,M.D. and Stampfer, M.D.,, Dr.P.H. , J.M. For the Dietary Intervention Randomized Controlled Trial (DIRECT) Group Weight Loss

with a Low-Carbohydrate, Mediterranean , or Low-Fat Diet: New Engl J Med 2008; 359:229- 241, July 2008.

42. Janet S. Hildebrand, MPH, American Cancer Society, Atlanta, Ga. Coffee, Tea, and Fatal Oral/Pharyngeal Cancer in a Large Prospective U.S. Cohort. Published online December 9, 2012 in the *American Journal of Epidemiology*.

43. Jensen, M.K., Koh-Baneijee P., Hu F.B., Franz, M., Sampson, L., Gronbaek M., Rimm E.B., Intakes of Whole grains, Beans and Grains and the Risk of Coronary Heart Disease in Men. American Journal of Clinical Nutrition, 2004 Dec. l80 (6): 1492-9.

44. Johnson R.K., Frary C. "Choose Beverages and Foods to Moderate Your Intake of Sugars: The 2000 Dietary Guidelines for Americans--What's All the Fuss About?" J Nutr. 2001 Oct;131(10):2766S-2771S.

45. Journal of the American Medical Association. "Caloric Sweetener Consumption and Dyslipidemia Among US Adults." Accessed April 20, 2010.

46. ISIC-The Institute for Scientific Information On Coffee,2019

47. Katzmanzyk, P.T, Church, T.S., Craig, C. L, and Bouchard, C. (2009). Sitting Time and Mortality from all Causes Cardiovascular Disease and Cancer. Medicine and Science in Sports and Exercise, 2009 May; 41 (5), 998-100.

48. Hall, Kevin D., PhD, Sachs, G., PhD, Chandramohen, D., BSc, Chow, C. C. PhD, Wang, Y,C,MD, Gortmaker, S. L., PhD, Swinburn B. A., MD, The Lancet Volume 378, Issue 9793, pages 826-837, August 2011.

49. Klem, M.L., Wing R.R., Chang C.H, Lang W., McGuire M.T., Sugerman H.J., Hutchison S.L, Makovich A.L. & Hill J.O. (2000). A Case Control Study of Successful Maintenance of a Substantial Weight Loss : Individuals Who Lost Weight

Through Surgery Versus Those Who Lost Weight Through Non-surgical Means. *International Journal of Obesity*, 24, 573-579.

50. Klem M.L., Wing R.R., McGuire M.T., Seagle H.M., & Hill J.O. (1997). A Descriptive Study of Individuals Successful at Long-term Maintenance of Substantial Weight Loss. *American Journal of Clinical Nutrition*, 66, 239-246.

51. Klem ML, Wing RR, McGuire MT, Seagle HM & Hill JO. (1998). Psychological Symptoms in Individuals Successful at Long-term Maintenance of Weight Loss. *Health Psychology*, 17, 336-345.

52. Klem M.L., Wing, R.R., Lang, W., McGuire, M.T. & Hill, J.O., (2000). Does Weight Loss Maintenance Become Easier Over Time? *Obesity Research*, 8, 438-444.

53. Lam, Michael, MD, Lam, Linking, J., Vitamin D and Cancer: The Vital Nutrient You Aren't Getting Enough of. ABAAHPFMNM,2019.

54. Lee I, Djoussé, L., Sesso H.D., Wang L., Buring J.E. Physical Activity and Weight Gain Prevention. JAMA. 2010; 303(12): 1173-1179.

55. Liu, S., Willett, W.C., Manson, J.E., Hu F.B., Rosner, B., Colditz, G. Relation Between Changes in Intakes of Dietary Fiber and Grain Products and Changes in Weight and Development of Obesity of Among Middle-aged Women. Am. J. Clin. Nutr. 2003;78:92.

56. Lopez-Garcia E.,Van Dam, R.M., Li T.Y., Rodriguesz-Artalejo F., Hu, F.B. The Relationship of Coffee Consumption with Mortality. *Ann Intern Med*. 2008; 148:904-914.

57. Maloney, Jennifer. Soda Loses US Crown: Americans Drink More Bottled Water, Wall Street Journal, March 9, 2017.

58. Condrasky, Marge, Ledke, J., Flood, Rolls, J., Barbara E. Chefs Opinion of Restaurant Portion Sizes. Obesity (2007) 15, 2086-2094.

59. McGuire M.T., Wing R.R., Hill J.O. (1999). The Prevalence of Weight Loss Maintenance Among American Adults. *International Journal of Obesity*, 23, 1314- 1319.

60. McGuire M.T., Wing, R.R., Klem, M.L., Hill, J.O. (1999). The Behavioral Characteristics of Individuals Who Lose Weight Unintentionally. *Obesity Research*, 7, 485-490.

61. McGuire M.T, Wing, R.R., Klem, M.L, Hill, J,O. (1999). Behavioral Strategies of Individuals who have Maintained Long-term Weight Losses. *Obesity Research*, 7, 334-341.

62. McGuire, M.T., Wing, R.R., Klem, M.L., Lang, W. & Hill, J.O. (1999). What Predicts Weight Regain Among a Group of Successful Weight Losers? *Journal of Consulting & Clinical Psychology*, 67, 177-185.

63. McGuire, MT, Wing, RR, Klem, ML, Seagle , HM & Hill, JO (1998). Long-term Maintenance of Weight Loss: Do People Who Lose Weight Through Various Weight Loss Methods Use Different Behaviors to Maintain Their Weight? *International Journal of Obesity*, 22, 572-577.

64. McKeown, N.M., Shea, Y.M., Jacques, M.K., Lichtenstein, P.F., Rogers, A.H., Booth, G., Saltzman E. Whole-grain Intake and Cereal Fiber are Associated with Lower Abdominal Adiposity in Older Adults. J Nutr 2009; 139; 1950-5.

65. l Lucas, Michel, O'Reilly, E, J., An Pan, M., Fariba, Willett, W. I., Okereke, C., Ascherio, O., Alberto. Coffee, Caffeine, and Risk of Completed Suicide: Results from Three Prospective Cohorts of American Adults. July 2014, Vol. 15, No. 5, Pages 377-386,

66. National Institutes of Health, Office of Dietary Supplements, and www: ods.od.nih. Gov/factsheets/calcium-Health Professional, PG. 1-16.

67. Neuhouser M.L., Wassertheil-Smoller, S., Thomson C., et al. (2009). "Multivitamin Use and Risk of Cancer and Cardiovascular Disease in the Women's Health Initiative Cohorts". *Arch Internal Medicine*, vol.169 No.3, February 9, 2009.

68. Neumark-Sztainer, D.M., Wall, J.Guo, S., Haines, M.J., and Eisenhberg, M., 2006 Obesity, Disordered Eating, and Eating Disorders in a Longitudinal Study of Adolescents: How Dieters Fare Five Years Later? J Amer Diet Assoc 106: 44) 559- 568.

69. Oldways' Mediterranean Diet Pyramid. (2009). Retrieved from, www.oldwayspt. Org

70. Osama, A., Mattila, E., Ermes, M., Van Gils, M., Wansink, B., & Korhonen, I., (2014) Weight Rhythms; Weight Increases During Weekends and Decreases During weekdays. Obesity Facts, 7 (DOI: 10.1159/000356147

71. P & G Personal Health Care Expert Views GI Health & Wellness Issue Six/ April 201

72. Schnatz, Peter, F., et al., Calcium/Vitamin D Supplementation, Serum 25-Hydroxyvitamin D Concentrations, and Cholesterol Profiles in the Women's Health Initiative Calcium/ Vitamin D Randomized Trial. *Menopause*, 2014; 1 DOI: 10.1097/GME.0000000000000188

73. Peterson, M., Gordon, Sen, A.P., Influence of Resistance Exercise on Lean Body Mass in Aging Adults Med Sci Sports Exercise, Feb 2011: 43 (2): 249-258

74. Phelan S, Wing, R.R., Hill J.O., Dibello J. (2003). Recovery from Relapse Among Successful Weight Maintainers. *American Journal of Clinical Nutrition*, 78, 1079-1084. Raynor H., Wing R.R., Phelan, S. (2005). Amount of Food Group

Variety Consumed in the Diet and Long-term Weight Loss Maintenance. *Obesity Research*, 13, 883-890.

75. Rideout T.C., Lun, B. Plant Sterols in the Management of Dyslipidemia in Patients with Diabetes. On the Cutting Edge. 2010; 31(6): 13-17.

76. *Rolls B.J.: The Volumetrics Eating Plan: Techniques and Recipes for Feeling Full on Fewer Calories. New York, HarperCollins Publishers Inc., 2005, pp. 8, 16–17.*

77. Rohsenow, D.J., Howland, J. The Role of Beverage Conegeners in Hangovers and Other Residual Effects of Alcohol Intoxication: A Review. J Current Drug Abuse Rev., 2010, June; 392076-9.

78. Rudolph, E., Faerbinger, K, Caffeine Intake From All Sources in Adolescents and Young Adults in Austria, Eur J Clin Nutr. 2014 Jul;68(7):793-8. doi: 10.1038/ejcn.2014.50. Epub 2014 Apr Shick, S.M., Wing, R.R., Klem M.L., McGuire, M.T., Hill, J.O. & Seagle, H.M.(1998). Persons Successful at Long-term Weight Loss and Maintenance Continue to Consume a Low Calorie, Low fat Diet. *Journal of the American Dietetic Association*, 98, 408-413.

79. Shilpa N., Bhupathiraju, A. P., Manson, J.E., Willett, W.W., Van Dam, R.M., Hu, F.M. "Changes in Coffee Intake and Subsequent Risk of Type 2 Diabetes: Three Large Cohorts of U.S. Men and Women," *Diabeteologia*, online April 24, 2014, DOI 10.1007/s00125-014-3235-7

80. 82.Sievart,Katherine: et al, Effect of Breakfast On Weight and Energy Intake; Systemic Review and Mata-analysis of Randomized Controlled Trials, BMJ 2019; 364:142.

81. Simkin-Silverman L.R., Wing R.R., Boraz, M.A., Kuller, L.H. Lifesyle Intervention Can Prevent Weight Gain During

Menopause; Results from a 5-year randomized Clinical Trial. Ann Behav Med 2003; Dec; 26 (3): 212-20.

82. Sofi F, Cesari F, Abbate, R., Gensini, G.F., Casini, A. (2008): Adherence to Mediterranean Diet and Health Statistics Meta-analysis BMJ (Clinical research ed.) 337 (Sept 11: 2): a1344.

83. Tomas, DePaulis, PhD. (2011, 02). Health Benefits of Coffee. *StudyMode.com.* Retrieved 02, 2011, from http://www.study-mode.com/essays/Health-Benefits-Of- Coffee-592030

84. Tree Nut Consumption and Weight management: A Scientific Review of the Literature. Michelle Wien, Dr.PH, RD, CDE & Joan Sabate, PhD, MD appeared in Summer 2011.

85. U.S. Department of Health and Human Services and U.S. Department of Agriculture. Dietary Guidelines for Americans, 2005. 6th Edition, Washington, DC: U.S. Government Printing Office, January 2005.

86. Ekelund, Ulf, et al., American Journal of Clinical Nutrition, April 2011 vol. 93 no.4, 826-835, Physical Activity and Weight Gain Prevention: Am Clinical Nutr 2011; 93(4) 826-835.

87. *Use of Nutritive and Nonnutritive Sweeteners, Volume 104, Issue 2, Pages 255- 275 (February 2004),* Journal of the Academy of Nutrition and Dietetics.

88. 87. Vegetarian Science Daily (April 21, 2008) reports that Carnegie Mellon researchers Christopher L.Weber and H. Scott Matthews say that shifting from an American diet to a vegetable-based one would reduce greenhouse gas emissions equivalent to driving 8,000 miles per year.

89. Wahlstrom, Kyla L. & Begalle, M. (1999). More Than Test Scores – Results of the Universal School Breakfast Pilot in Minnesota. *Topics in Clinical Nutrition,* vol 15: no 1. Jan 31, 2019.

90. Walton, Alice G. For Weight Loss, Breakfast May Not Be The Most Important Meal of the Day, Healthcare. Jan. 31,2019.

91. Weight Loss with a Low-Carbohydrate, Mediterranean, or Low-Fat Diet: New Engl. J. Med 2008; 359:229-241, July 2008.

92. D. Wikoff, What You Need to Know About Mercury in Fish and Shellfish, 2004 EPA and FDA Advice For: Women Who Might Become Pregnant, Women Who are Pregnant, Nursing Mothers, Young Children.

93. Wells, Jeffrey, Study: Men are Primary Grocery Shoppers In US Households, 7/28/2017.

94. Wells, Jeffrey. Smartphones to Store Transformations: 6 Grocery Trends to Watch in 2019.

95. Wing, R.R., & Hill J.O. (2001). Successful Weight Loss Maintenance. *Annual Review of Nutrition*, 21, 323-341.

96. Wyatt ,H.R., Grunwald, G.K., Seagle, H.M., Klem, M.L., McGuire, M.T., Wing, R.R., & Hill, J.O. (1999). Resting Energy Expenditure in Reduced-Obese Subjects in the National Weight Control Registry. *American Journal of Clinical Nutri-tion*, 69, 1189-1193.

97. Wyatt, H.R., Grunwald, O.K., Mosca, C.L., Klem, M.L., Wing, R.R., Hill, J.O., (2002). Long- term Weight Loss and Breakfast in Subjects in the National Weight Control Registry. *Obesity Research*, 10, 78-82.

98. Wyatt, H.R., Phelan, S, Wing, R.R., Hill,J.O., (2005). Lessons from Patients Who Have Successfully Maintained Weight Loss. *Obesity Management*, 1, 56-61.

99. Probiotics linked to Weight Loss in Obese, Overweigh. Health News Article News for Physicians and Medical Professionals January 2018

100. Wan et. al Journal Gut 'High Fat diet, Low Carb Diet May Create Microbiome Changes to the Gut that Could Lead to Metabolic Disorders in Young Adults.

101. Krautkamer, K.A, ,et. Al, Diet= Microbiota Interactions Mediate Global Epigenetic Programming in Multiple Host Tissues

102. Molecular Cell doi:10, 1016/j.molcel.2016, 10. 025, published online 23, November 2016

103. Shivam, Joshi, MD[1,2;] Robert J. Ostfeld, R.J.,MD, MSc3; Michelle McMacken, MD[1,2,] Ketogenic Diet for Obesity and Diabetes-Enthusiasm Outpaces Evidence. JAMA, 2019:321 (11) : 1081-1093

104. Shivam Joshi, MD[1,2;] Robert J. Ostfeld, MD, MSc3; Michelle McMacken,, MD[1,2] JAMA, 2019:321 (11) : 1081-1093

105. Victor N. Zhang, PhD et al, Association of Dietary Cholesterol or Egg Consumption with Incident of Cardiovascular Disease and Mortality

106. Zee, Kristi Here's An Easy Hack For Keeping Portion Control in Check When Dining Out, Cooking Lite, October 12, 2018.

107. WSJ, Tuesday, JUNE9, 2020, R9 A multipronged Strategy for Obesity by Laura Landro.

108. https://www.heart.org/en/healthy-living/healthy-eating/eat-smart/sugar/how-much-sugar-is-too-much - 238k - Cached - Similar pages

109. https://foodandnutrition.org/blogs/stone-soup/sugar-bad-cancer-patients

110. Fairlife.com

111. www.wsj.com/articles/men-urged-to-limit-alcohol-to-one-drink-a-day-amid-new-concerns-11597688916

112. https://www.tommys.org/pregnancy-information/about-us/tommys-midwives-blog/tommys-responds-news-about-consuming-caffeine-during-pregnancy

113. WSJ. New Limits Urged on American's Sugar Consumption Amid Rising Obesity Concerns, 9/28/2020.

114. www.Cardiosmart.org: Focus on Healthy Fats Instead of Saturated Fat Limits, Research Suggests.

115. www. Oldways Webinar 1/27/2021: Unlocking the Cardiovascular Benefits of Tea

116. ArTzEoLr9QW2h47hnGAm-3AGiving Up Alcohol in the Era of Covid19

117. ATeFHccfKTyGhk1zg9gGzBAMediterranean Diet Recipes For Healthy Aging

ACKNOWLEDGEMENTS

Writing a book takes more than the work of the authors. It takes the cooperation of people sharing their support and talents to put together the final product.

We would like to thank the following people:

Our families for tolerating the time we spent on working on this project. And for the messy kitchen and dining room tables covered with computers, papers, and pens.

Debra Mae Funderwhite, the book photographer for designing the book cover.

Amit Dey and Soumi Goswami, graphic artists for putting our book together in a prompt and professional manner.

Carol Taylor, registered dietitian and editor who worked with us to put together a new edition of our book. It was especially helpful to not only have an editor work with us, but also a registered dietitian who knows our language.

Chris Smith, Arlington Heights Memorial Library Librarian who helped us during the Covid-19 lockdown to provide help and support.

Brad Johnson, author and search engine optimizer for formatting the book during the Covid-19 lockdown providing us with his excellent support.

Our special gratitude goes out to our thousands of patients and clients we have provided nutrition counseling to over the years. Without them, there would be no Too Busy to Diet.

Thank you and happy, healthy eating.

Jackie and Monica

ABOUT THE AUTHORS

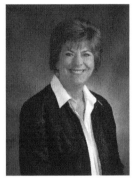

Jacqueline King is a registered dietitian/nutritionist, Certified Diabetes Care & Education Specialist and Fellow in the Academy of Nutrition and Dietetics. She has worked at Rush University Medical Center, Chicago, Il. and Northwestern Memorial Hospital, Chicago, Il. where she worked as the Research Dietitian at the Diabetes in Pregnancy Center. She received her Bachelor Degree in Medical Dietetics at University of Illinois at Chicago and her Master's Degree in Food and Nutrition at Northern Illinois University in Dekalb, Il.

She is working as a consulting dietitian seeing patients and working with corporations. Her hobbies include: reading voraciously, exercising, traveling, sewing, socializing with family and friends, and exploring ethnic foods.

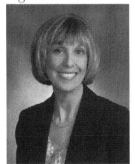

Monica Joyce is a registered dietitian/nutritionist, and Certified Diabetes Care & Education Specialist. She received her Bachelor's Degree in Foods and Nutrition at Mundelein College/Loyola University in Chicago, Il. She received her Master's Degree in Human Services Administration at Spertus College, Chicago, Il.

Monica is working as a diabetes educator at Lake Forest Northwestern, Lake Forest, Il. She is also a partner with an endocrinologist in the company Culinary Medics.

Monica is passionate about helping people make healthy choices and enjoying these choices. She enjoys traveling, trying new recipes/foods and sharing these with her family.

- For bulk copies of Too Busy to Diet for employers, member groups, health clubs, gyms, health related companies, health or fitness classes, businesses, educational classes or personal use please send an email to: dietking1@comcast.net
- For individualized nutrition plans and consultation contact : dietking1@comcast.net

Thanks for reading our book. If you enjoyed this book and found it useful, please leave an honest review at Amazon.com

Check out our blog at www.toobusytodietbook.com. Leave questions and topics of interest.

NOTES

Made in the USA
Columbia, SC
13 May 2022

60392570R00193